Breeding Fantasy

Erotic Pregnancy Play

Carrie Bellyfull

ISBN: 9781778905476
Imprint: Telephasic Workshop
Copyright © 2024 Carrie Bellyfull.
All Rights Reserved.

Contents

Introduction   1
Understanding Breeding Fantasy   1

Creating the Fantasy   25
Building a Safe and Consensual Relationship   25

Bibliography   33
Roleplaying Scenarios   48

Safety and Health Considerations   121
Physical Health   121
Mental and Emotional Well-being   139

Beyond the Bedroom: Integrating Breeding Fantasy into Daily Life   163
Communication and Consent   163
Fantasy Enhancement Techniques   179

Ethical Considerations and Conclusion   203
Consent and Boundaries Revisited   203
The Future of Breeding Fantasy   217

Index   233

Introduction

Understanding Breeding Fantasy

Defining the concept

Breeding fantasy, often referred to as erotic pregnancy play, is a complex and multifaceted phenomenon that intertwines sexual desire with the themes of reproduction and pregnancy. This section will delve into the various dimensions of breeding fantasy, aiming to provide a comprehensive understanding of its definition, significance, and implications within the realm of erotic roleplay.

Understanding Breeding Fantasy

At its core, breeding fantasy encompasses a desire for conception, pregnancy, and the associated experiences that come with them. This desire can manifest in various ways, from the simple act of fantasizing about impregnation to engaging in elaborate roleplay scenarios that simulate the entire process of conception and gestation.

The appeal of breeding fantasies lies in their ability to evoke strong emotional and psychological responses. For many, the idea of creating life can be intensely erotic, tapping into primal instincts and biological drives. The interplay of vulnerability, intimacy, and power dynamics often found in these fantasies adds another layer of complexity that can heighten the experience.

Theoretical Framework

To better understand breeding fantasy, it is essential to consider several theoretical frameworks that inform our understanding of human sexuality and desire. The following theories offer valuable insights:

- **Biological Determinism:** This theory posits that human behavior, including sexual desire, is largely influenced by biological factors such as hormones and reproductive instincts. Breeding fantasies may stem from an innate drive to procreate, reflecting deep-seated evolutionary urges.

- **Psychosexual Development:** Sigmund Freud's theories on psychosexual development suggest that early experiences shape adult sexual desires. Breeding fantasies could be linked to unresolved conflicts or desires from childhood, particularly those relating to family, nurturing, and sexuality.
- **Social Constructivism:** This perspective emphasizes the role of societal norms and cultural narratives in shaping sexual desires. Breeding fantasies may be influenced by cultural representations of motherhood, femininity, and masculinity, as well as societal attitudes towards sexuality and reproduction.
- **Feminist Theory:** Feminist perspectives on sexuality challenge traditional notions of gender roles and power dynamics. Breeding fantasies can be analyzed through the lens of feminist theory, exploring how they reflect or subvert societal expectations of gender, motherhood, and sexuality.

Historical Context

The historical context of breeding fantasy reveals much about societal attitudes toward sexuality and reproduction. Throughout history, various cultures have celebrated fertility and motherhood, often intertwining these themes with eroticism.

In ancient societies, fertility rites and rituals were common, celebrating the life-giving power of women. These practices often included elements of eroticism, linking sexuality and reproduction in ways that resonate with modern breeding fantasies.

However, as societal norms evolved, so too did the perception of sexuality and reproduction. The rise of the sexual liberation movement in the 20th century began to challenge traditional views on sex and reproduction, allowing for a broader exploration of sexual desires, including those related to breeding fantasies.

Taboos and Controversies

Despite the increasing acceptance of diverse sexual practices, breeding fantasies remain shrouded in taboo. Societal attitudes toward pregnancy, motherhood, and sexuality often create a complex web of stigma and controversy.

Critics may argue that breeding fantasies perpetuate harmful stereotypes about women and motherhood, reducing women to mere vessels for reproduction.

Additionally, concerns regarding consent and the potential for coercion in breeding scenarios can complicate discussions around the fantasy.

It is crucial to approach these topics with sensitivity and a commitment to understanding the nuances of individual desires. Engaging in open dialogue about breeding fantasies can help dismantle the stigma surrounding them and promote a more inclusive understanding of human sexuality.

Importance of Consent and Boundaries

In any exploration of breeding fantasy, the principles of consent and boundaries are paramount. Engaging in roleplay scenarios that involve pregnancy and reproduction necessitates clear communication and mutual agreement between partners.

Establishing consent protocols and discussing boundaries before engaging in breeding play is essential to ensure that all parties feel safe and respected. This process may include discussing potential triggers, emotional responses, and the specific dynamics of the roleplay scenario.

Moreover, the use of safewords and regular check-ins during roleplay can help maintain a sense of safety and control, allowing participants to navigate the emotional complexities of breeding fantasies with care.

Psychological Appeal of Pregnancy Play

The psychological appeal of breeding fantasy can be attributed to several factors:

- **Desire for Connection:** Many individuals are drawn to breeding fantasies due to the deep emotional connection they can foster between partners. The act of creating life can symbolize intimacy, trust, and vulnerability, enhancing the erotic experience.

- **Exploration of Identity:** Engaging in breeding fantasies allows individuals to explore different aspects of their identity, including gender roles, sexuality, and parental desires. This exploration can lead to personal growth and self-discovery.

- **Power Dynamics:** Breeding fantasies often involve elements of dominance and submission, allowing individuals to explore power dynamics within their relationships. This exploration can be thrilling and liberating, providing a safe space to navigate complex emotions.

- **Fantasy as Escape:** For some, breeding fantasies serve as a form of escapism, providing an opportunity to step outside the constraints of everyday life.

The allure of pregnancy and reproduction can create a fantasy world where individuals can explore their deepest desires without judgment.

Types of Roleplay Scenarios

Breeding fantasies can manifest in various roleplay scenarios, each offering unique opportunities for exploration and expression. Some common scenarios include:

- **Natural Conception:** Roleplaying scenarios that simulate the experience of natural conception, often focusing on the excitement and anticipation surrounding the act.

- **Fertility Exploration:** Engaging in roleplay that centers around fertility, ovulation, and the desire to conceive, allowing partners to explore their fantasies related to reproductive health.

- **Medical Play:** Incorporating elements of medical fetishism into breeding fantasies, such as roleplaying doctor-patient scenarios that explore insemination techniques or fertility treatments.

- **Postpartum Dynamics:** Exploring the emotional and physical aspects of postpartum recovery, allowing partners to navigate the complexities of motherhood and sexuality.

Communication and Negotiation

Effective communication and negotiation are essential components of engaging in breeding fantasies. Partners should feel comfortable discussing their desires, boundaries, and any concerns that may arise during roleplay.

This process may involve:

- **Open Dialogue:** Encouraging honest conversations about individual fantasies and desires, fostering a sense of trust and understanding.

- **Setting Boundaries:** Clearly defining what is acceptable and what is not within the context of breeding play, ensuring that all parties feel safe and respected.

- **Regular Check-Ins:** Establishing a system for ongoing communication during roleplay, allowing partners to address any discomfort or emotional triggers that may arise.

In conclusion, breeding fantasy is a rich and complex area of exploration within erotic roleplay. By understanding its definition, historical context, psychological appeal, and the importance of consent and communication, individuals can engage in breeding fantasies in a safe and fulfilling manner. As we continue to explore the intricacies of human sexuality, it is essential to approach these topics with an open mind and a commitment to understanding the diverse desires that shape our erotic experiences.

Historical background

Breeding fantasy and erotic pregnancy play have deep roots in human sexuality, intertwined with the evolution of societal norms, cultural beliefs, and individual desires. Understanding the historical context of these fantasies requires us to examine the interplay between sexuality, reproduction, and the social constructs that surround them.

Throughout history, the concept of fertility has been both revered and fetishized. In many ancient cultures, fertility was synonymous with prosperity and abundance. The worship of fertility deities, such as the Roman goddess Venus or the Egyptian goddess Hathor, reflects a societal reverence for the ability to conceive and bear children. These figures were often depicted in art and literature as embodiments of sexual allure and motherhood, intertwining eroticism with the sanctity of reproduction.

The historical discourse surrounding pregnancy has also been shaped by various philosophical and medical theories. For instance, during the Enlightenment, the emergence of rational thought led to a more scientific understanding of reproduction. Thinkers like René Descartes and later, Charles Darwin, began to explore the biological aspects of reproduction, laying the groundwork for modern reproductive science. However, this scientific progress did not eliminate the eroticization of pregnancy; rather, it added layers of complexity to how society perceives and engages with the concept of breeding.

In the 19th century, the Victorian era marked a significant shift in attitudes toward sexuality and reproduction. While the era is often characterized by sexual repression, it also gave rise to a fascination with the female body and its reproductive capabilities. The idea of the "angel in the house" idealized motherhood, while simultaneously creating a dichotomy between sexual desire and maternal virtue. This tension contributed to the emergence of breeding fantasies, as individuals sought to reconcile their sexual urges with societal expectations.

The 20th century witnessed a dramatic transformation in attitudes toward sexuality, particularly with the advent of the sexual revolution in the 1960s and

1970s. This period challenged traditional norms and embraced sexual liberation, allowing individuals to explore their desires more openly. The feminist movement also played a crucial role in redefining women's relationships with their bodies and reproductive choices. This newfound freedom fostered an environment where breeding fantasies could flourish, as individuals began to articulate and explore their desires without the constraints of societal judgment.

In contemporary society, breeding fantasy has gained visibility through various media, including literature, film, and online communities. The rise of the internet has facilitated the formation of niche communities where individuals can share their fantasies and experiences related to pregnancy play. This digital landscape has allowed for greater exploration of the psychological and emotional dimensions of breeding fantasies, as participants engage in discussions about consent, boundaries, and the complexities of desire.

Despite this increased visibility, breeding fantasies remain a topic of controversy and taboo. Critics often raise concerns about the potential for non-consensual dynamics, coercion, and the fetishization of pregnancy in ways that may undermine women's autonomy. It is essential to navigate these discussions with sensitivity, emphasizing the importance of consent and communication in all aspects of erotic roleplay.

Moreover, the psychological appeal of breeding fantasies can be understood through various theoretical lenses. Psychoanalytic theory, particularly the works of Sigmund Freud, posits that sexual desires often stem from unconscious drives and conflicts. Breeding fantasies may represent a manifestation of deeper psychological needs, such as the desire for intimacy, nurturing, or power exchange. Additionally, attachment theory suggests that individuals may seek out breeding fantasies as a way to explore their relational dynamics and desires for connection.

In summary, the historical background of breeding fantasy reveals a complex interplay between societal norms, cultural beliefs, and individual desires. From ancient fertility rituals to contemporary erotic roleplay, the fascination with pregnancy has evolved, reflecting broader changes in attitudes toward sexuality and reproduction. As we delve into the intricacies of breeding fantasy, it is crucial to acknowledge this historical context and approach the subject with an understanding of the diverse perspectives and experiences that shape it.

Taboos and controversies

Breeding fantasies and erotic pregnancy play exist at the intersection of desire and societal norms, often challenging conventional boundaries. These themes evoke a spectrum of reactions, ranging from intrigue to discomfort, and are steeped in various taboos that warrant exploration. Understanding these taboos not only deepens the appreciation of such fantasies but also illuminates the broader societal attitudes towards sexuality, reproduction, and gender roles.

Cultural Perspectives on Pregnancy

Pregnancy is often revered as a natural and beautiful state; however, it is also heavily laden with societal expectations and norms. In many cultures, pregnancy is idealized, viewed as a rite of passage, yet simultaneously, it is shrouded in shame and stigma when associated with sexual desire. The duality of pregnancy as both a sacred and sexualized experience creates a complex landscape for those who wish to explore breeding fantasies.

For instance, in some cultures, the act of conceiving is celebrated, while in others, it may evoke feelings of guilt or anxiety, especially when viewed through the lens of non-traditional relationships or sexual practices. The taboo surrounding the enjoyment of pregnancy as a sexual fantasy can be traced to deeply rooted beliefs about motherhood and femininity, which often prioritize the nurturing aspect over the sexual.

Gender Dynamics and Power Structures

The discussion of breeding fantasies cannot occur without acknowledging the gender dynamics at play. Historically, women's sexuality has been policed, and their reproductive capabilities have been a source of both power and oppression. In many societies, women are expected to embody the archetype of the nurturing mother, which can conflict with their desires for sexual agency and exploration.

Breeding fantasies often involve power dynamics that can be both empowering and problematic. The fantasy may allow participants to explore dominance and submission, where the act of breeding becomes a metaphor for control and ownership. This power exchange can be thrilling, yet it also raises ethical questions about consent and coercion. For instance, a partner may fantasize about being "taken" or "bred," which can blur the lines of consent if not carefully negotiated.

The Controversy of Consent

Consent is a cornerstone of any erotic fantasy, yet the nature of breeding play can complicate this principle. The fantasy of impregnation often evokes the notion of permanence and consequence, which can lead to concerns about coercion and the potential for emotional harm. Participants must navigate the delicate balance between fantasy and reality, ensuring that all parties are fully informed and consenting to the roleplay.

Moreover, societal views on consent in relation to reproductive rights further complicate this issue. The historical context of women's autonomy over their bodies has evolved, but remnants of control and ownership linger. Engaging in breeding fantasies can evoke feelings of guilt, especially if they challenge personal beliefs about reproduction and motherhood.

Ethical Considerations in Roleplay

The ethical considerations surrounding breeding fantasies extend beyond consent. Participants must also consider the implications of their roleplay on their relationships and personal lives. Engaging in breeding fantasies can lead to misunderstandings if partners are not aligned in their desires. For example, one partner may view the fantasy as a mere roleplay, while the other may develop genuine feelings or expectations about pregnancy and parenting.

Additionally, the portrayal of pregnancy in media and popular culture often reinforces stereotypes and unrealistic expectations. Participants in breeding fantasies may inadvertently perpetuate harmful narratives that equate a woman's worth with her ability to conceive. It is essential to approach these fantasies with sensitivity and awareness of the broader societal implications.

Navigating Social Stigma

The societal stigma surrounding breeding fantasies can lead to feelings of isolation and shame for those who wish to explore them. Many individuals fear judgment from peers or family members, which can inhibit open discussions about desires and boundaries. This stigma can be particularly pronounced for individuals who identify as part of the LGBTQ+ community, where traditional narratives about reproduction may not apply.

To navigate this stigma, individuals may seek out supportive communities or engage in anonymous online forums where they can share experiences and insights without fear of judgment. Building a network of like-minded individuals can provide a sense of belonging and validation, allowing for healthier explorations of breeding fantasies.

Conclusion

In conclusion, the taboos and controversies surrounding breeding fantasies and erotic pregnancy play are multifaceted, encompassing cultural, gender, ethical, and social dimensions. Engaging with these themes requires a nuanced understanding of the underlying beliefs and attitudes that shape our perceptions of sexuality and reproduction. By fostering open communication, establishing consent, and addressing societal stigma, individuals can explore these fantasies in a safe and fulfilling manner, ultimately enriching their sexual experiences and personal growth.

Importance of Consent and Boundaries

In the realm of erotic roleplay, particularly in breeding fantasies, the concepts of consent and boundaries are not merely guidelines; they are the very foundation upon which safe and fulfilling experiences are built. Consent serves as the cornerstone of any intimate encounter, ensuring that all parties involved are willing participants who understand the implications of their choices. This section delves into the multifaceted importance of consent and boundaries within breeding fantasies, exploring the theoretical underpinnings, potential problems, and practical examples that illustrate their significance.

Theoretical Framework of Consent

Consent, in its most basic form, is the agreement between individuals to engage in a specific activity. According to the *Encyclopedia of Sexuality*, consent must be informed, voluntary, and revocable at any time. This aligns with the principles outlined by the *World Health Organization*, which states that consent is not simply a yes or no but a continuous dialogue throughout any sexual encounter.

In breeding fantasies, where the themes of reproduction and pregnancy are central, the stakes can feel particularly high. The psychological appeal of these fantasies often intertwines with deep-seated desires for intimacy, connection, and even the exploration of power dynamics. Therefore, understanding consent within this context requires a nuanced approach that acknowledges the emotional and psychological layers involved.

Defining Boundaries

Boundaries are the limits that individuals set regarding what they are comfortable with in any relationship or interaction. Establishing clear boundaries is essential in breeding fantasies, as it allows individuals to articulate their desires, fears, and limits openly. According to *Esther Perel*, boundaries create a safe space for exploration, enabling partners to engage in fantasies without fear of crossing into discomfort or harm.

Potential Problems and Misunderstandings

One of the most significant challenges in the realm of consent and boundaries is the potential for misunderstandings. In breeding play, where the themes can evoke strong emotions and complex feelings, miscommunication can lead to situations where one partner feels violated or uncomfortable. For instance, if one partner expresses a desire to roleplay a scenario involving conception without explicitly discussing boundaries, the other partner may assume that they are comfortable with all aspects of that scenario, leading to potential emotional distress.

Moreover, societal taboos surrounding pregnancy and reproduction can further complicate the conversation about consent. Individuals may feel pressured to conform to certain expectations or norms, leading them to agree to scenarios they are not genuinely comfortable with. This highlights the importance of ongoing communication and check-ins throughout the roleplay experience.

Practical Examples of Consent and Boundaries in Breeding Fantasies

To illustrate the importance of consent and boundaries, consider the following practical examples:

- **Scenario 1: The Initial Discussion**
  Before engaging in any breeding fantasy, partners should have an open dialogue about their desires and limits. For instance, one partner may express a desire to explore the excitement of trying to conceive, while the other may have concerns about the emotional implications of such a roleplay. By discussing these feelings openly, both partners can establish a clear understanding of what is acceptable and what is not.

- **Scenario 2: Establishing Safewords**
  During the roleplay, partners should agree on safewords that can be used to pause or stop the scene if discomfort arises. For example, if one partner feels overwhelmed during a particularly intense moment, they could use a pre-agreed safeword to signal that they need a break. This practice reinforces the idea that consent is an ongoing process, not a one-time agreement.

- **Scenario 3: Aftercare and Emotional Support**
  Aftercare is a crucial component of any intimate experience, particularly in breeding fantasies where emotions can run high. After the roleplay, partners should engage in a debriefing conversation to discuss what worked, what didn't, and how they felt throughout the experience. This not only helps to reinforce boundaries but also fosters intimacy and trust between partners.

Conclusion

In conclusion, the importance of consent and boundaries in breeding fantasies cannot be overstated. These elements serve as the bedrock for safe and enjoyable experiences, allowing individuals to explore their desires while respecting each other's limits. By fostering open communication, establishing clear boundaries, and engaging in ongoing dialogues about consent, partners can create a fulfilling and enriching environment for their erotic roleplay. Ultimately, the journey into breeding fantasies can be a profound exploration of intimacy, power dynamics, and personal growth, but it must be navigated with care, respect, and a steadfast commitment to consent.

The psychological appeal of pregnancy play

Pregnancy play, a niche yet captivating aspect of erotic roleplay, is steeped in psychological complexity. Understanding the underlying motivations can illuminate why this fantasy resonates with many individuals. The allure of pregnancy play can be dissected through various psychological lenses, including desire for intimacy, power dynamics, and the exploration of taboo.

Desire for Intimacy

At its core, pregnancy play often symbolizes a profound connection between partners. The act of creating life is inherently intimate, and for many, roleplaying pregnancy can evoke feelings of closeness and bonding. This intimacy is not merely physical; it encompasses emotional vulnerability and trust. The psychological theory of attachment, as proposed by Bowlby (1969), suggests that strong emotional bonds are crucial for human development. In the context of pregnancy play, individuals may seek to replicate the nurturing and protective aspects of attachment, allowing them to explore their desires for closeness in a safe environment.

Power Dynamics

Pregnancy play also taps into the intricate web of power dynamics that exists within sexual relationships. The concept of dominance and submission is prevalent in many erotic fantasies, and pregnancy play is no exception. The roles can be fluid, with one partner embodying the dominant figure—often taking on the role of the 'breeder'—while the other assumes a more submissive position, embracing the vulnerability associated with pregnancy.

The psychological framework of BDSM, as discussed by Dossie Easton and Janet W. Hardy in *The New Topping Book* (2013), emphasizes the importance of consent and negotiation in establishing power dynamics. In pregnancy play, the dynamic can shift as the fantasy unfolds; the submissive partner may experience the thrill of surrendering control, while the dominant partner revels in the responsibility of guiding the experience. This interplay can lead to heightened arousal and satisfaction, as both partners explore their fantasies within the bounds of mutual consent.

Exploration of Taboo

Another significant element contributing to the psychological appeal of pregnancy play is the exploration of taboo. Pregnancy, as a natural biological process, is often surrounded by societal norms and expectations. Engaging in pregnancy play allows individuals to challenge these norms, creating a space where they can confront and redefine their perceptions of sexuality and reproduction.

Freud's theory of repression suggests that societal taboos can lead to the intensification of desire. When individuals engage in fantasies that break social conventions, such as pregnancy play, they may experience a rush of excitement and liberation. This thrill can be both exhilarating and fulfilling, as it allows participants to step outside the confines of their everyday lives and explore their desires without fear of judgment.

Psychological Theories and Models

To further understand the psychological appeal of pregnancy play, we can consider several theoretical models. The *Cognitive-Behavioral Theory* posits that our thoughts, beliefs, and attitudes shape our behaviors. In the context of pregnancy play, individuals may develop specific cognitive schemas that associate pregnancy with pleasure, intimacy, and power. These schemas can reinforce the desire to engage in roleplay scenarios that reflect these themes.

Additionally, the *Erotic Fantasy Theory* suggests that sexual fantasies serve as a means of exploring desires that may be difficult to express in reality. Pregnancy play can provide a safe outlet for individuals to navigate their feelings about parenthood, sexuality, and intimacy. As individuals engage in these fantasies, they may experience catharsis, allowing them to confront underlying anxieties or desires related to reproduction and relationships.

Examples of Psychological Appeal

Consider the following examples that illustrate the psychological appeal of pregnancy play:

1. **Intimacy and Connection**: A couple may engage in pregnancy roleplay as a way to foster intimacy. By creating scenarios where one partner 'becomes' pregnant, they can explore the emotional aspects of nurturing and support, deepening their bond.

2. **Power Exchange**: In another scenario, a dominant partner may guide their submissive through the experience of pregnancy play, emphasizing control and care. This dynamic can heighten arousal, as the submissive partner embraces their vulnerability while the dominant partner assumes a protective role.

3. **Breaking Taboos**: A participant may find excitement in roleplaying scenarios that challenge societal norms, such as exploring non-traditional family structures or the idea of pregnancy outside of conventional relationships. This exploration can serve as a form of rebellion against societal expectations, leading to a sense of empowerment.

Conclusion

The psychological appeal of pregnancy play is multifaceted, intertwining themes of intimacy, power dynamics, and the exploration of taboo. By understanding these underlying motivations, individuals can engage in pregnancy play with greater awareness and intention, fostering a deeper connection with their partners while navigating the complexities of desire. As with any fantasy, the key lies in open communication, consent, and mutual exploration, allowing for a fulfilling and enriching experience that honors the desires of all involved.

Exploring the power dynamics

Power dynamics in breeding fantasy and erotic pregnancy play are multifaceted and can manifest in various ways, influencing the experiences of those involved. Understanding these dynamics is crucial for engaging in this type of roleplay safely and consensually. This section will explore the theoretical underpinnings of power exchange, the implications of these dynamics in breeding fantasy, and practical examples to illustrate these concepts.

Theoretical Framework

At the core of power dynamics in erotic roleplay lies the concept of *power exchange*, which is often rooted in BDSM practices. Power exchange refers to the deliberate transfer of power from one individual (the submissive) to another (the dominant) within a consensual context. This transfer can enhance intimacy and trust, creating a safe space for exploring fantasies. In the context of breeding fantasy, power dynamics can be particularly pronounced, as they often involve themes of control, fertility, and reproduction.

Dominance and Submission Dominance and submission (D/s) relationships are characterized by a clear delineation of roles, with one partner taking on a more dominant role while the other assumes a submissive position. In breeding scenarios, the dominant partner may take control over the conception process, while the submissive partner may express a desire to be "filled" or to experience pregnancy. This dynamic can evoke feelings of vulnerability and safety for the submissive, while the dominant partner may feel empowered by their ability to fulfill the fantasy.

The Role of Consent Consent is paramount in any exploration of power dynamics, particularly in breeding fantasy. Both partners must communicate their desires, boundaries, and limits before engaging in roleplay. The use of safewords and ongoing check-ins can help maintain a sense of safety and security, allowing both partners to explore their fantasies without fear of crossing boundaries. It is essential to establish a mutual understanding of what power exchange means within the context of breeding play, ensuring that both partners feel respected and valued.

Implications of Power Dynamics in Breeding Fantasy

The implications of power dynamics in breeding fantasy are vast and can lead to various emotional and psychological responses. Understanding these implications can help participants navigate their experiences more effectively.

Emotional Vulnerability Engaging in breeding fantasy often requires a significant degree of emotional vulnerability. The submissive partner may experience feelings of exposure and dependence, while the dominant partner may feel an increased sense of responsibility. This emotional vulnerability can enhance intimacy between partners, but it can also lead to discomfort if not managed properly. Open communication about feelings and experiences during and after roleplay is essential for addressing any emotional challenges that may arise.

Exploring Control and Trust   Breeding fantasies often involve themes of control, both in terms of the physical act of conception and the emotional landscape of the relationship. The dominant partner may exert control over the submissive's body, which can be thrilling for both parties. However, this control must be tempered with trust; the submissive must trust that their partner will respect their boundaries and prioritize their well-being. Establishing trust is crucial for creating a safe environment where both partners can explore their desires without fear of harm.

Practical Examples

To illustrate the complexities of power dynamics in breeding fantasy, consider the following scenarios:

Scenario 1: Natural Conception Roleplay   In a natural conception roleplay, the dominant partner takes on the role of a "fertilizer," while the submissive partner embodies a "willing vessel." The dominant partner may dictate the timing and circumstances of the act, while the submissive partner surrenders control, expressing their desire to conceive. This dynamic can heighten the thrill of the experience, as both partners engage in a dance of power and submission. However, it is essential to establish clear boundaries regarding the fantasy's emotional and physical implications.

Scenario 2: Medical Play and Artificial Insemination   In a more clinical setting, the roleplay may involve artificial insemination, where the dominant partner assumes the role of a medical professional. The submissive partner may be portrayed as a patient seeking to conceive. This scenario can incorporate elements of medical fetishism, with the dominant partner wielding power through knowledge and expertise. The submissive partner's vulnerability is heightened, as they rely on the dominant partner to guide them through the process. Again, consent and communication are vital to ensure that both partners feel comfortable and respected throughout the experience.

Scenario 3: Breeding Contracts and Rituals   Some individuals may choose to create breeding contracts or rituals that outline the terms of their roleplay. These documents can serve as a tangible representation of the power dynamics at play, reinforcing the commitment to consent and boundaries. The dominant partner may take the lead in drafting the contract, while the submissive partner reviews and negotiates its terms. This process can deepen the sense of trust and collaboration between partners, allowing them to explore their fantasies within a structured framework.

Navigating Challenges

While exploring power dynamics in breeding fantasy can be exhilarating, it also presents challenges. Participants must be aware of potential pitfalls and take proactive steps to address them.

Addressing Power Imbalances Power imbalances can arise in any relationship, particularly in D/s dynamics. It is crucial for both partners to recognize and address these imbalances to ensure a healthy and consensual experience. Regular check-ins and discussions about feelings can help mitigate any discomfort that may arise from perceived inequalities in power.

Red Flags and Emotional Triggers Participants should be vigilant for red flags that may indicate an unhealthy dynamic, such as coercion or manipulation. Additionally, emotional triggers related to past experiences may surface during roleplay. Open communication about these triggers is essential for maintaining a safe and supportive environment.

Conclusion

Exploring the power dynamics inherent in breeding fantasy can lead to profound experiences of intimacy, trust, and pleasure. By understanding the theoretical foundations of power exchange, recognizing the implications of these dynamics, and navigating challenges with care, partners can create a fulfilling and consensual space for their fantasies. Ultimately, the key to a successful breeding fantasy lies in the commitment to open communication, mutual respect, and a shared understanding of boundaries.

Types of Roleplay Scenarios

Roleplay scenarios in the realm of breeding fantasy can be as varied and nuanced as the individuals who engage in them. Each scenario can evoke different emotions, dynamics, and experiences, allowing participants to explore the depths of their fantasies while maintaining a focus on safety and consent. Below, we delve into several prominent types of roleplay scenarios, examining their psychological implications, potential challenges, and illustrative examples.

1. Natural Conception

Natural conception scenarios often center around the excitement and intimacy of trying to conceive a child. This type of roleplay can involve a variety of settings, from a romantic evening at home to a spontaneous encounter in a more adventurous location.

Psychological Implications: The thrill of natural conception roleplay can evoke feelings of vulnerability and trust, as participants navigate the intimate act of creating life together. This scenario may tap into the deep-seated desires for connection, nurturing, and the primal instinct to reproduce.

Challenges: Participants must communicate openly about their desires and boundaries, ensuring that both partners feel comfortable with the scenario. It is crucial to address any potential emotional triggers related to fertility or past experiences.

Example: A couple might set the scene with romantic music and dim lighting, engaging in passionate foreplay that culminates in a deliberate attempt to conceive. They might use props such as ovulation kits or fertility charts to heighten the sense of realism.

2. Fertility and Ovulation Exploration

This scenario focuses on the biological aspects of conception, emphasizing the science behind fertility and ovulation. Participants can roleplay as a couple exploring their reproductive health, discussing ovulation cycles, and engaging in acts designed to increase the likelihood of conception.

Psychological Implications: Engaging in this type of roleplay can foster a sense of empowerment and knowledge about one's body, while also enhancing intimacy through shared learning experiences.

Challenges: It is essential to ensure that both partners are on the same page regarding their comfort with discussing reproductive health, as this can be a sensitive topic for some.

Example: A couple could create a scenario where they research fertility together, using educational materials to discuss the ovulation cycle, and then transitioning into intimate activities that align with the fertile window.

3. The Excitement of Trying to Conceive

This scenario captures the anticipation and thrill associated with the process of trying to conceive. Participants can roleplay the emotional highs and lows of this journey, from the excitement of potential pregnancy to the anxiety of waiting for results.

Psychological Implications: The emotional rollercoaster of this scenario can strengthen the bond between partners, as they navigate the shared experience of hope and longing.

Challenges: It is vital to establish clear boundaries to prevent feelings of disappointment or frustration from impacting the relationship.

Example: A couple might roleplay the moment of taking a pregnancy test, creating a narrative around the anticipation of the results, and celebrating or comforting each other based on the outcome.

4. Intimacy During Pregnancy

This scenario allows couples to explore the dynamics of intimacy during pregnancy, focusing on the physical and emotional changes that occur. Participants can roleplay as expectant parents, navigating the complexities of their evolving relationship.

Psychological Implications: Intimacy during pregnancy can evoke a sense of nurturing and protection, fostering deeper emotional connections between partners.

Challenges: Participants should communicate openly about their comfort levels with physical touch and intimacy, as pregnancy can bring about various physical and emotional changes.

UNDERSTANDING BREEDING FANTASY

Example: Couples might engage in gentle, affectionate touch, focusing on the growing belly and discussing their hopes and dreams for their future child, creating a safe space for vulnerability.

5. Fantasizing About Labor and Birth

Roleplaying labor and birth can be an intense and transformative experience, allowing participants to explore the raw power of creation. This scenario can involve various elements, from the physical sensations of labor to the emotional support provided by a partner.

Psychological Implications: This type of roleplay can evoke feelings of empowerment and strength, as participants navigate the challenges of bringing new life into the world.

Challenges: Participants must be mindful of the emotional weight of this scenario, as it can bring up feelings related to personal experiences with childbirth or loss.

Example: A couple might create a birthing scene, using props such as birthing balls or blankets, and roleplay the supportive dynamics of a partner assisting through labor, emphasizing communication and encouragement.

6. Postpartum Roleplay and Recovery

Postpartum roleplay focuses on the period following childbirth, exploring themes of recovery, bonding with the newborn, and the evolving dynamics of the couple's relationship.

Psychological Implications: This scenario can help participants process the complexities of postpartum emotions, including joy, anxiety, and the challenges of new parenthood.

Challenges: It is crucial to approach this scenario with sensitivity, recognizing that postpartum experiences can vary widely and may include feelings of vulnerability or inadequacy.

Example: Participants could roleplay a scene where they navigate the challenges of new parenthood, discussing the joys and struggles of caring for a newborn while supporting each other emotionally.

7. Artificial Insemination

Artificial insemination roleplay allows couples to explore the medical and emotional aspects of conception through assisted reproductive technologies. Participants can roleplay as a couple undergoing the insemination process, discussing their hopes and fears.

Psychological Implications: This scenario can evoke feelings of hope and anticipation, as well as anxiety related to the uncertainties of fertility treatments.

Challenges: It is essential to communicate openly about any personal experiences with fertility treatments, as this can be a sensitive topic for many.

Example: A couple might set the scene in a medical environment, discussing the steps involved in artificial insemination while engaging in intimate activities that symbolize their commitment to starting a family.

8. Breeding as a Power Exchange

Breeding fantasies often incorporate elements of power exchange, where one partner takes on a dominant role while the other assumes a submissive position. This dynamic can enhance the thrill of the scenario, adding layers of complexity to the experience.

Psychological Implications: The interplay of dominance and submission can heighten arousal and deepen emotional connections, allowing participants to explore their desires in a safe and consensual manner.

Challenges: It is crucial to establish clear boundaries and safewords, ensuring that both partners feel secure in their roles throughout the experience.

Example: A dominant partner might guide their submissive through a breeding scenario, emphasizing control and surrender, while incorporating elements of aftercare and emotional support.

9. Creating Breeding Contracts and Rituals

Incorporating contracts and rituals into breeding roleplay can add a layer of commitment and seriousness to the fantasy. Participants can create personalized agreements that outline their desires, boundaries, and expectations.

Psychological Implications: This scenario can foster a sense of security and trust, as both partners actively participate in shaping their experience.

Challenges: It is essential to regularly revisit and renegotiate contracts, ensuring that both partners feel comfortable and fulfilled in their roles.

Example: A couple might draft a playful contract that outlines their breeding fantasies, incorporating elements of humor and creativity while emphasizing the importance of consent and communication.

10. Breeding Communities and Events

Exploring breeding fantasies within the context of communities and events can provide opportunities for connection and shared experiences. Participants can engage with like-minded individuals, attending workshops or gatherings focused on breeding play.

Psychological Implications: Being part of a community can enhance feelings of belonging and validation, allowing participants to explore their fantasies in a supportive environment.

Challenges: Navigating societal judgment and stigma may be a concern, requiring participants to establish boundaries regarding privacy and discretion.

Example: Couples might attend a breeding-themed event, participating in discussions and activities that foster connection and exploration of their shared interests.

Conclusion

In conclusion, the variety of roleplay scenarios within breeding fantasy offers a rich tapestry of experiences for participants to explore. By understanding the psychological implications and challenges associated with each scenario, individuals can create fulfilling and consensual experiences that deepen their connections and enhance their intimacy. As with any form of roleplay, clear communication, consent, and emotional support are paramount to ensuring a positive and enriching experience.

Communication and negotiation

Effective communication and negotiation are foundational components in any intimate relationship, especially when exploring complex fantasies such as breeding play. This section delves into the theoretical underpinnings of communication, the potential challenges that may arise, and practical examples to illustrate how to navigate these discussions.

Theoretical Framework

Communication theory posits that effective interaction relies on clarity, mutual understanding, and active listening. According to the *Transactional Model of Communication*, both parties are simultaneously senders and receivers of messages, which emphasizes the importance of feedback in ensuring comprehension. This model is particularly relevant in the context of erotic roleplay, where nuances of consent, desire, and boundaries must be clearly articulated.

$$C = f(S, R, M, F) \qquad (1)$$

Where:

- C = Communication effectiveness
- S = Sender's clarity
- R = Receiver's understanding
- M = Message content
- F = Feedback mechanism

Challenges in Communication

1. **Fear of Judgment**: Individuals may hesitate to express their desires due to fear of being judged or misunderstood. This apprehension can lead to a lack of openness, stifling the exploration of fantasies.

2. **Differing Levels of Interest**: Partners may have varying degrees of interest in breeding play. One partner might be enthusiastic, while the other feels ambivalent. This disparity necessitates careful negotiation to ensure both parties feel comfortable and valued.

3. **Misinterpretation of Signals**: Non-verbal cues can be misread, leading to misunderstandings. For example, a partner's silence may be interpreted as agreement when it might actually indicate discomfort or uncertainty.

4. **Cultural and Societal Influences**: Societal norms surrounding pregnancy and sexuality can create additional layers of complexity. Individuals may struggle to reconcile their fantasies with societal expectations, leading to internal conflict.

Strategies for Effective Communication

1. **Establishing a Safe Space**: Create an environment conducive to open dialogue. This may involve choosing a comfortable setting, free from distractions, where both partners feel secure to express their thoughts.

2. **Utilizing "I" Statements**: Encourage the use of "I" statements to express feelings and desires without placing blame. For example, instead of saying, "You never want to talk about my fantasies," one might say, "I feel anxious when we don't discuss my interests."

3. **Active Listening**: Practice active listening by acknowledging and reflecting back what the other person has said. This not only shows respect but also clarifies understanding. For instance, "What I hear you saying is that you're not comfortable with the idea of artificial insemination, is that correct?"

4. **Setting Boundaries**: Clearly outline personal boundaries and preferences. This can be done through discussions about what each partner is willing to explore and what is off-limits. A boundary-setting exercise could look like this:

- List three things you are excited to explore.

- List three things you are uncomfortable with.

- Discuss how you can both feel safe and fulfilled within these parameters.

5. **Negotiation Techniques**: Engage in a collaborative negotiation process to arrive at mutually satisfying scenarios. This may include brainstorming different roleplay scenarios, discussing the emotional implications, and agreeing on safe words or signals to use during play.

Practical Examples

1. **Scenario Exploration**: Imagine two partners, Alex and Jamie, who are interested in exploring breeding fantasies. They might begin by discussing their individual interests in the fantasy. Alex expresses a desire to roleplay natural conception, while Jamie is more interested in the emotional aspects of pregnancy.

> Alex: "I really want to explore the thrill of trying to conceive together. It excites me to think about the intimacy involved in that process."
>
> Jamie: "I love that idea, but I also want to make sure we're addressing the emotional side of it, like how we would feel if we were actually pregnant."

Through this dialogue, they can negotiate a scenario that includes both elements, ensuring that both partners feel engaged and respected.

2. **Feedback Mechanism**: During their roleplay, Alex and Jamie agree to check in with each other regularly. They establish a system where they pause after significant moments to discuss feelings and comfort levels, which helps them navigate any discomfort that may arise.

> Jamie: "Let's take a moment. How are you feeling about what just happened?"
>
> Alex: "I'm feeling really excited, but I want to make sure we're still on the same page."

3. **Addressing Discomfort**: If at any point Jamie feels overwhelmed, they can use a predetermined safe word, such as "pineapple," to pause the scene and discuss what's bothering them. This practice reinforces the importance of consent and emotional safety.

Conclusion

Communication and negotiation are not merely transactional; they are transformative processes that can deepen intimacy and trust within a relationship. By approaching discussions about breeding fantasies with openness and empathy, partners can create a rich tapestry of shared experiences that honor both individual desires and collective boundaries. The key lies in fostering an environment where both partners feel empowered to express their fantasies, negotiate their limits, and ultimately explore the depths of their erotic imaginations together.

Creating the Fantasy

Building a Safe and Consensual Relationship

Establishing trust and communication

Establishing trust and communication is foundational to any intimate relationship, especially when exploring the nuanced and often sensitive realm of breeding fantasy and erotic pregnancy play. This section delves into the theories surrounding trust, the common challenges faced, and practical strategies for effective communication, ensuring that all parties feel safe and respected.

Theoretical Frameworks

Trust is often defined as the reliance on the integrity, strength, ability, or character of a person or entity. In the context of erotic roleplay, trust encompasses emotional safety, vulnerability, and the assurance that boundaries will be respected. According to Rempel et al. (1985), trust can be broken down into three dimensions:

- **Predictability:** The extent to which one can anticipate the actions of their partner based on past interactions.

- **Dependability:** The belief that one's partner will act in a way that is supportive and respectful of their needs.

- **Faith:** A deeper level of trust that goes beyond rational assessment, often tied to emotional bonds.

Building trust requires time and consistent positive interactions, particularly when navigating the complexities of breeding fantasies.

Common Challenges

While the desire to explore breeding fantasies can be exciting, it can also introduce challenges, such as:

- **Fear of Judgment:** Individuals may worry about being judged for their desires, leading to reluctance in sharing their fantasies.
- **Misunderstandings:** Without clear communication, partners may misinterpret intentions or desires, leading to conflict.
- **Vulnerability:** Engaging in intimate roleplay can make individuals feel exposed, which can inhibit open dialogue.
- **Power Imbalances:** In some dynamics, one partner may feel less empowered to express their needs or boundaries, complicating communication.

Strategies for Effective Communication

To foster trust and enhance communication, consider the following strategies:

1. **Open Dialogue:** Initiate conversations about desires, boundaries, and any concerns regarding breeding fantasy. Use "I" statements to express feelings without placing blame. For example, "I feel excited about exploring this fantasy, but I also have some concerns about how we approach it."

2. **Active Listening:** Ensure that both partners practice active listening, which involves fully concentrating on what the other is saying, rather than formulating a response while they speak. Reflect back what you hear to confirm understanding. For instance, "What I hear you saying is that you're excited but also apprehensive about the idea of pregnancy play. Is that correct?"

3. **Regular Check-ins:** Establish a routine for checking in with each other about feelings and experiences related to the roleplay. This can be done before, during, and after play sessions. Use open-ended questions to facilitate deeper discussions, such as "How did you feel during our last session?"

4. **Establishing Boundaries:** Clearly define what is acceptable and what is not. This can involve discussing hard limits (non-negotiable boundaries) and soft limits (areas that require negotiation). It may also be beneficial to create a written agreement that outlines these boundaries.

BUILDING A SAFE AND CONSENSUAL RELATIONSHIP

5. **Utilize Safewords:** Implement safewords to signal when a partner is uncomfortable or needs to pause the roleplay. Safewords can be simple (e.g., "red" for stop, "yellow" for slow down) and should be respected without question.

6. **Emotional Support:** Understand that engaging in breeding fantasies can evoke a range of emotions. Providing emotional support during and after roleplay can enhance trust. Discuss aftercare rituals that may include cuddling, talking about the experience, or simply being present with one another.

7. **Normalize Vulnerability:** Acknowledge that vulnerability is a part of intimacy. Create an environment where both partners feel safe to express fears and insecurities without judgment.

Examples in Practice

Consider a couple, Alex and Jamie, who are exploring breeding fantasies. They begin by having an open conversation about their interests. Alex expresses a desire to roleplay a scenario involving natural conception, while Jamie shares concerns about the implications of such a fantasy.

> Alex: "I'm really interested in trying out a scenario where we explore the excitement of trying to conceive. How do you feel about that?"

Jamie responds with their feelings, highlighting both excitement and apprehension. They agree to set boundaries around the roleplay and establish a safeword for any discomfort that may arise. After their first roleplay session, they check in with each other to discuss what worked and what didn't, reinforcing their commitment to open communication.

Conclusion

Establishing trust and communication is not merely a precursor to engaging in breeding fantasies; it is an ongoing process that enriches the relationship. By fostering a safe space for dialogue, partners can explore their desires with confidence, ultimately enhancing intimacy and connection. Remember, the journey into erotic pregnancy play should be as pleasurable and fulfilling as the fantasies themselves, grounded in mutual respect and understanding.

Setting boundaries and limits

In the realm of breeding fantasy and erotic pregnancy play, establishing boundaries and limits is a crucial aspect of ensuring a safe and enjoyable experience for all parties involved. Boundaries serve as the framework within which individuals can explore their desires while maintaining a sense of security and respect for one another. This section will delve into the theory behind boundaries, common challenges that may arise, and practical examples to guide you in setting effective limits.

Theoretical Framework of Boundaries

Boundaries can be understood through the lens of interpersonal communication theory, which emphasizes the importance of clear and open dialogue in relationships. According to [Brown(2010)], boundaries are not merely restrictions; they are essential components of healthy relationships that define where one person ends, and another begins. They help individuals articulate their needs, desires, and limits, fostering an environment of trust and respect.

The concept of boundaries can be categorized into several types:

- **Physical Boundaries:** These pertain to personal space and physical touch. In the context of breeding fantasy, this may include discussing what types of physical interaction are acceptable during roleplay.

- **Emotional Boundaries:** These involve the emotional safety of individuals. It is crucial to communicate feelings and emotional triggers that could arise during the exploration of pregnancy themes.

- **Time Boundaries:** This refers to the duration and timing of roleplay sessions. Setting limits on how long a scene will last can help prevent emotional exhaustion.

- **Material Boundaries:** These relate to the use of props, costumes, or toys during roleplay, ensuring that all participants are comfortable with the items involved.

Common Challenges in Setting Boundaries

Despite the importance of boundaries, individuals may face several challenges when attempting to establish them:

- **Fear of Judgment:** Individuals may worry about being judged for their desires or limits, leading to reluctance in expressing their needs.

- **Miscommunication:** Without clear communication, misunderstandings can occur, resulting in discomfort or harm.

- **Evolving Desires:** As experiences unfold, individuals may discover new limits or desires, necessitating ongoing discussions about boundaries.

- **Power Dynamics:** In BDSM and kink scenarios, power dynamics may complicate boundary-setting, as one partner may feel pressured to acquiesce to the other's desires.

Practical Steps for Setting Boundaries

To effectively set boundaries and limits, consider the following practical steps:

1. Open Dialogue Initiate a conversation with your partner(s) about boundaries well before engaging in roleplay. Use open-ended questions to encourage dialogue, such as:

> "What are your thoughts on the types of scenarios we might explore together?"

2. Identify Personal Limits Encourage each participant to reflect on their personal limits. This can be facilitated through a pre-roleplay questionnaire that addresses various aspects of the fantasy, including:

- What aspects of pregnancy are appealing?

- Are there any specific scenarios that feel uncomfortable or off-limits?

- How do you feel about incorporating medical play?

3. Establish Safewords Creating a safeword is an essential part of boundary-setting. A safeword is a predetermined term that, when spoken, indicates the need to pause or stop the roleplay. Common examples include:

- **Red:** Stop immediately.

- **Yellow:** Slow down or check-in.

- **Green:** Everything is okay; continue.

4. Regular Check-Ins During roleplay, make it a practice to check in with each other. This can be as simple as asking, "How are you feeling right now?" This practice reinforces emotional safety and demonstrates care for one another's well-being.

5. Reevaluate Boundaries Post-Roleplay After a session, engage in a debriefing conversation to discuss what worked and what didn't. This can help identify any new boundaries or adjustments that may be necessary for future encounters.

Examples of Setting Boundaries

To illustrate the process of setting boundaries, consider the following hypothetical scenarios:

Scenario 1: Discussing Physical Touch In a breeding fantasy roleplay, one partner expresses a desire for intimate physical touch, while the other is uncomfortable with certain forms of contact. They engage in a conversation to clarify acceptable touch:

> Partner A: "I love the idea of being intimate during our roleplay, but I want to ensure we're both comfortable. Can we talk about what kinds of touch are okay?" Partner B: "Absolutely! I'm okay with kissing and cuddling, but I'd prefer to avoid anything too intense."

Scenario 2: Emotional Triggers During a roleplay session, one partner realizes that a specific scenario triggers feelings of anxiety related to past experiences. They pause the roleplay to communicate their discomfort:

> Partner A: "I'm feeling a bit overwhelmed with this scenario. Can we switch to something else?" Partner B: "Of course! Let's take a moment and talk about what would feel better for you."

Scenario 3: Evolving Desires After several roleplay sessions, one partner discovers a newfound interest in a specific aspect of breeding fantasy. They bring it up during a check-in:

> Partner A: "I've been thinking about how we roleplay, and I'm curious about exploring more medical aspects. How do you feel about that?" Partner B: "I'm open to it! Let's discuss what that might look like."

Conclusion

Setting boundaries and limits is a vital component of engaging in breeding fantasy and erotic pregnancy play. By fostering open communication, identifying personal limits, establishing safewords, and regularly checking in with one another, participants can create a safe and pleasurable environment for exploration. Remember that boundaries are not static; they evolve with experience and understanding. Embrace the journey of discovery together, and prioritize the emotional and physical well-being of all involved.

Bibliography

[Brown(2010)] Brown, B. (2010). *The Gifts of Imperfection: Let Go of Who You Think You're Supposed to Be and Embrace Who You Are.* Hazelden Publishing.

Safewords and check-ins

In the realm of breeding fantasy and erotic pregnancy play, the establishment of safewords and regular check-ins is paramount to ensuring a safe, consensual, and enjoyable experience for all parties involved. This section delves into the significance of safewords, how to implement them effectively, and the importance of check-ins during roleplay scenarios.

Understanding Safewords

Safewords are predetermined words or signals that participants can use to pause, stop, or alter the course of a scene. They serve as a vital communication tool, especially in scenarios that may evoke intense emotions or physical sensations. The concept of safewords is rooted in the principles of consent and respect, emphasizing that all parties retain the right to withdraw from the experience at any moment.

Choosing Effective Safewords

When selecting safewords, it is crucial to choose terms that are easy to remember and unlikely to be confused with typical conversation. Common practices include:

- **Traffic Light System:** This system uses three colors to denote different levels of comfort:
    - **Green:** Everything is good; continue.
    - **Yellow:** Slow down or check in; something feels off.

- **Red:** Stop immediately; the scene must end.

+ **Unique Words:** Choose words that are unlikely to arise during the play, such as "pineapple" or "unicorn." This minimizes confusion and ensures clarity.

Implementing Safewords in Roleplay

Once safewords have been established, it is essential to communicate their meaning and use to all participants. Here are some strategies for effective implementation:

1. **Pre-Scene Discussion:** Before engaging in roleplay, discuss the safewords openly. Ensure that everyone understands their significance and agrees to respect them.

2. **Practice Scenarios:** Engage in a practice scene where safewords are utilized, allowing participants to become comfortable using them in a low-stakes environment.

3. **Reinforcement:** During the roleplay, periodically remind participants of the safewords, especially if the scene becomes intense or emotionally charged.

The Importance of Check-Ins

Check-ins are integral to maintaining a safe space during roleplay. They involve pausing periodically to assess the emotional and physical well-being of all participants. Regular check-ins can prevent misunderstandings and ensure that everyone is enjoying the experience.

When to Check-In

Consider implementing check-ins at the following intervals:

+ **Before Starting:** Assess how each participant is feeling and confirm consent.

+ **During Intense Moments:** Pause during particularly intense scenes to gauge comfort levels.

+ **After Major Scene Changes:** Following significant shifts in the roleplay dynamic, check in to ensure everyone remains comfortable.

How to Conduct Check-Ins

Check-ins should be conducted in a manner that fosters open communication. Here are some effective techniques:

1. **Ask Open-Ended Questions:** Encourage participants to express their feelings by asking questions like, "How are you feeling right now?" or "Is there anything you'd like to change?"

2. **Use Non-Verbal Signals:** For scenarios where verbal communication may be challenging, establish non-verbal signals (e.g., a thumbs up for "good" or a hand wave for "stop").

3. **Create a Safe Space for Feedback:** Encourage participants to share their thoughts and feelings without fear of judgment. This can be facilitated by establishing a culture of respect and understanding.

Addressing Potential Problems

Despite best efforts, challenges may arise during roleplay. Here are common issues and strategies for addressing them:

- **Miscommunication:** If a participant feels uncomfortable but does not vocalize it, it may lead to distress. Encourage an environment where all feelings are valid and promote the use of safewords without hesitation.

- **Emotional Triggers:** Participants may encounter unexpected emotional triggers. Regular check-ins can help identify these triggers early, allowing for adjustments in the scene.

- **Power Dynamics:** In scenarios involving dominance and submission, the submissive partner may feel pressured to continue despite discomfort. Reinforcing the use of safewords and regular check-ins can help mitigate this risk.

Conclusion

In summary, the use of safewords and check-ins is essential in breeding fantasy and erotic pregnancy play. By establishing clear communication channels and prioritizing the emotional and physical well-being of all participants, individuals can explore their fantasies in a safe, consensual, and fulfilling manner. Embracing these practices not only enhances the experience but also fosters deeper connections and trust between partners, ultimately enriching the erotic journey.

Emotional support and aftercare

Emotional support and aftercare are crucial components of engaging in breeding fantasy and erotic pregnancy play. Aftercare refers to the practices and processes that follow a scene or roleplay, intended to help participants transition back to their everyday lives while ensuring their emotional and psychological well-being. This section explores the significance of aftercare, its various forms, and the theoretical frameworks that support its necessity.

The Importance of Aftercare

Aftercare serves several essential functions in the context of breeding fantasy:

- **Emotional Regulation:** Engaging in intense roleplay can evoke strong emotions, including joy, vulnerability, fear, or anxiety. Aftercare provides a space for participants to process these emotions, helping them to regulate and understand their feelings.

- **Reinforcement of Trust:** Aftercare reinforces the trust established between partners. By attending to each other's emotional needs post-roleplay, partners demonstrate their commitment to each other's well-being, fostering a deeper connection.

- **Facilitating Communication:** Aftercare encourages open dialogue about the experience. Participants can discuss what they enjoyed, what was challenging, and any feelings that arose during the scene, leading to better understanding and future experiences.

Forms of Aftercare

Aftercare can take many forms, and it is essential to tailor these to the preferences and needs of the individuals involved. Some common forms include:

- **Physical Comfort:** This may involve cuddling, gentle touch, or providing a safe space for relaxation. Physical affection can be grounding and reassuring, helping to ease any residual tension from the roleplay.

- **Verbal Reassurance:** Partners can engage in conversations that affirm their feelings for each other, express gratitude for the experience, and validate each other's emotions. Phrases like "I'm here for you" or "You did amazing" can be particularly comforting.

- **Reflection and Debriefing:** This involves discussing the roleplay in detail, sharing thoughts and feelings about the experience, and addressing any concerns that may have arisen. This debriefing process can help clarify boundaries and preferences for future encounters.

- **Engaging in Calming Activities:** Activities such as watching a favorite movie, taking a walk, or enjoying a warm bath together can help participants transition back to their everyday selves and provide a sense of normalcy after an intense experience.

Theoretical Frameworks

Understanding the psychological implications of aftercare can be enhanced through various theoretical frameworks:

- **Attachment Theory:** This theory posits that secure attachment styles are crucial for healthy relationships. Aftercare can reinforce secure attachments by providing reassurance and fostering emotional intimacy, which is particularly important in the context of breeding fantasies that may involve vulnerability.

- **Polyvagal Theory:** This theory emphasizes the role of the autonomic nervous system in emotional regulation. Aftercare can help regulate physiological responses to stress and anxiety, promoting a sense of safety and calmness post-roleplay.

- **Trauma-Informed Care:** Recognizing that some participants may have past traumas that could be triggered during roleplay, aftercare becomes essential in providing a safe space for healing and support, ensuring that all participants feel secure and respected.

Examples of Aftercare Practices

Implementing effective aftercare practices can vary widely between individuals and scenarios. Here are some examples:

- **Creating a Safe Space:** Designate a specific area where aftercare can take place, filled with comforting items like blankets, pillows, and soft lighting to create a nurturing environment.

- **Using Comfort Items:** Encourage the use of comfort items, such as stuffed animals or favorite blankets, to help soothe participants after intense roleplay.

- **Journaling:** Encourage participants to journal their thoughts and feelings after the roleplay. This can facilitate self-reflection and provide an outlet for processing emotions.

- **Check-in Rituals:** Establish a routine for checking in with each other after roleplay sessions, allowing for ongoing communication about feelings and experiences.

Conclusion

Emotional support and aftercare are indispensable components of engaging in breeding fantasy and erotic pregnancy play. By prioritizing aftercare, participants can ensure that their experiences are not only pleasurable but also emotionally enriching, fostering deeper connections and promoting psychological well-being. As with all aspects of roleplay, clear communication, consent, and understanding each other's needs are paramount in creating a fulfilling and safe environment for exploration.

Consent protocols and negotiations

In the realm of breeding fantasy and erotic pregnancy play, establishing clear consent protocols and engaging in thorough negotiations is paramount. This process not only ensures the safety and comfort of all parties involved but also enhances the overall experience by fostering trust and intimacy. This section delves into the essential components of consent protocols, the negotiation process, and the importance of maintaining an open dialogue.

Defining Consent

Consent is a mutual agreement between participants to engage in specific activities. It is crucial that consent is:

- **Informed:** All parties must have a clear understanding of what they are consenting to, including the nature of the activities, potential risks, and emotional implications.

- **Freely Given:** Consent should be provided without any form of coercion, manipulation, or pressure. Participants must feel empowered to say no at any point.

- **Reversible:** Consent can be withdrawn at any time, and participants should feel comfortable doing so without fear of repercussions.
- **Specific:** Consent should be specific to the activities being discussed. A broad agreement does not imply consent for all actions.

The Importance of Negotiation

Negotiation is the process through which participants discuss their desires, boundaries, and expectations before engaging in breeding fantasy scenarios. This is an opportunity for individuals to express their fantasies, explore limits, and establish a mutual understanding of what will occur during the roleplay.

- **Identifying Desires:** Each participant should articulate their desires and interests within the breeding fantasy. This includes discussing what aspects of pregnancy play they find appealing, whether it involves natural conception, artificial insemination, or other scenarios.
- **Discussing Boundaries:** It is essential to establish clear boundaries regarding what is acceptable and what is off-limits. This may include physical boundaries, emotional triggers, and any topics that may cause discomfort.
- **Creating Safewords:** A safeword is a predetermined word or signal that participants can use to pause or stop the roleplay if they feel uncomfortable or wish to reassess the situation. Safewords should be easy to remember and distinct from regular conversation.

Examples of Consent Protocols

To illustrate the importance of consent protocols, consider the following hypothetical scenarios:

> **Example**
>
> **Scenario 1:** Alex and Jamie are discussing a breeding fantasy that involves natural conception. They agree on a safeword, "red," to indicate when either feels overwhelmed. During their roleplay, Jamie suddenly feels uncomfortable with the direction the fantasy is taking. By using the safeword, they pause the scene, allowing for a discussion about boundaries and feelings before proceeding.

> **Example**
>
> **Scenario 2:** Taylor and Morgan are exploring artificial insemination roleplay. During their negotiation, Taylor expresses a desire to incorporate medical play elements. Morgan, however, has a boundary regarding medical scenarios due to past trauma. They negotiate an alternative scenario that satisfies both parties without crossing Morgan's limits.

Addressing Common Problems

Despite best intentions, issues may arise during the negotiation process. It is essential to be aware of potential problems and address them proactively:

- **Miscommunication:** Participants may interpret desires and boundaries differently. To mitigate this, it is crucial to ask clarifying questions and ensure mutual understanding.

- **Power Dynamics:** In some relationships, one partner may hold more power, which can complicate the negotiation process. It is vital to create an environment where all parties feel equal and empowered to voice their needs.

- **Emotional Triggers:** Participants may have unrecognized emotional triggers related to pregnancy or conception. Discussing these openly before engaging in roleplay can help prevent unexpected discomfort.

Ongoing Communication

Consent and negotiation are not one-time events; they require ongoing communication. Participants should regularly check in with each other, both during and after roleplay sessions. This practice helps to reinforce trust and ensures that both parties feel safe and respected.

- **Post-Scene Discussions:** After a roleplay session, take time to discuss what worked well and what could be improved. This feedback loop is essential for growth and understanding.

- **Reevaluating Boundaries:** As individuals explore their fantasies, their boundaries may shift. Regularly revisiting consent protocols allows participants to adapt to these changes.

Conclusion

Consent protocols and negotiations are foundational to engaging in breeding fantasy and erotic pregnancy play. By prioritizing clear communication, mutual understanding, and ongoing dialogue, participants can create a safe and fulfilling environment for exploration. Remember, the journey of discovery in breeding fantasies is most rewarding when all parties feel respected, heard, and empowered to express their desires and boundaries.

Dealing with societal judgment and stigma

In the realm of breeding fantasy and erotic pregnancy play, societal judgment and stigma can pose significant challenges for individuals and couples who seek to explore these desires. This section delves into the complexities of societal perceptions, the psychological impact of stigma, and strategies for managing external judgments while fostering a fulfilling and consensual exploration of breeding fantasies.

Understanding Societal Judgment

Societal judgment refers to the negative evaluations or criticisms that individuals may face from their communities, families, or peers regarding their sexual preferences and practices. Breeding fantasies, often considered taboo, can evoke strong reactions due to cultural norms surrounding sexuality, reproduction, and femininity. The stigma associated with these fantasies can be understood through several theoretical lenses:

1. **Social Constructionism:** This theory posits that societal norms and values shape our understanding of acceptable behavior. Breeding fantasies challenge conventional views on sexuality and reproduction, leading to potential ostracization from mainstream society.

2. **Labeling Theory:** According to this theory, individuals who engage in non-normative sexual practices may be labeled as deviant. This labeling can lead to a self-fulfilling prophecy, where individuals internalize negative perceptions and experience feelings of shame or guilt.

3. **Cultural Norms:** Many cultures uphold rigid definitions of sexuality, often valorizing reproductive heterosexuality while demonizing alternative expressions. Breeding fantasies may be viewed as excessive or abnormal, further entrenching stigma.

Psychological Impact of Stigma

The psychological effects of societal judgment can be profound. Individuals may experience:
 - Shame and Guilt: The fear of being judged can lead to feelings of shame regarding one's desires. This internal conflict can diminish sexual satisfaction and hinder open communication with partners.
 - Isolation: Stigmatization can result in social isolation, as individuals may feel compelled to hide their fantasies from friends and family, leading to a lack of support and understanding.
 - Anxiety and Stress: The pressure to conform to societal expectations can create anxiety, impacting overall mental health and well-being. The constant fear of judgment can hinder individuals from fully embracing their desires.

Strategies for Managing Societal Judgment

1. **Building a Supportive Community:** Connecting with like-minded individuals through online forums, local meetups, or kink events can provide a sense of belonging. Engaging with communities that celebrate diverse sexual expressions can help mitigate feelings of isolation.

2. **Education and Advocacy:** Educating oneself and others about breeding fantasies can challenge misconceptions. Sharing knowledge about the importance of consent, safety, and emotional well-being can foster understanding and acceptance.

3. **Open Communication with Partners:** Establishing a safe space for dialogue with partners about desires and boundaries can strengthen relationships. Discussing societal pressures openly can help partners navigate external judgments together.

4. **Reframing Internal Narratives:** Challenging negative self-talk and reframing thoughts about one's desires can be empowering. Affirmations and self-compassion practices can help individuals embrace their fantasies without shame.

5. **Engaging with Mental Health Professionals:** Seeking support from therapists who specialize in sexual health can provide valuable insights and coping strategies. Therapy can help individuals process feelings of shame and develop healthier relationships with their desires.

Examples of Navigating Societal Judgment

Consider the case of Alex and Jamie, a couple exploring breeding fantasies. Initially, they faced societal judgment from friends who held traditional views on relationships and reproduction. To cope, they sought out online communities where they found validation and support. By participating in discussions and sharing experiences, they learned to embrace their desires without fear.

Another example is Sarah, who felt ashamed of her breeding fantasies. After attending a workshop on sexual empowerment, she learned to communicate openly with her partner. They established a safe word and discussed boundaries, allowing Sarah to explore her desires in a supportive environment. Over time, she reframed her narrative, recognizing that her fantasies were a natural expression of her sexuality.

Conclusion

Dealing with societal judgment and stigma in breeding fantasy and erotic pregnancy play requires resilience and self-acceptance. By fostering supportive communities, engaging in open communication, and challenging societal norms, individuals can navigate the complexities of their desires. Ultimately, embracing one's fantasies within a consensual and safe framework can lead to a more fulfilling and liberated sexual experience.

Managing privacy concerns

In the realm of breeding fantasy and erotic pregnancy play, managing privacy concerns is paramount. Engaging in such intimate and often taboo scenarios can expose individuals to societal judgment and personal vulnerability. Therefore, understanding the implications of privacy and developing strategies to protect oneself and one's partner is essential for a fulfilling and safe experience.

The Importance of Privacy

Privacy serves as a protective barrier, safeguarding personal information, fantasies, and experiences from unwanted scrutiny. In the context of breeding fantasy, where themes of reproduction and intimacy are explored, the stakes are particularly high. The fear of social stigma can inhibit individuals from fully embracing their desires. According to [?], the relationship between power and knowledge plays a significant role in how individuals navigate their sexual identities. Keeping fantasies private allows individuals to reclaim autonomy over their narratives, free from external judgment.

Common Privacy Concerns

Several privacy concerns may arise when engaging in breeding fantasy:

- **Disclosure of Personal Information:** Sharing sensitive information about one's fantasies or experiences can lead to unintended exposure. This may include revealing personal identities, locations, or specific details about one's relationship dynamics.

- **Digital Footprint:** In an increasingly digital world, online discussions and interactions can leave a lasting footprint. Engaging in forums or social media can inadvertently expose individuals to unwanted attention or harassment.

- **Judgment from Peers and Family:** The potential for negative judgment from friends and family can create a barrier to open communication about one's desires. This concern can lead to feelings of isolation and shame, which may hinder the exploration of fantasies.

- **Consent of Partners:** When engaging in breeding fantasies, it is crucial to consider the privacy of all parties involved. Partners may have different comfort levels regarding what to share or keep private, necessitating clear communication and mutual agreement.

Strategies for Managing Privacy

To effectively manage privacy concerns, individuals can adopt several strategies:

1. **Establish Clear Boundaries:** Before engaging in breeding fantasy scenarios, partners should discuss and establish clear boundaries regarding what information can be shared and with whom. This conversation can help prevent misunderstandings and ensure that both parties feel secure.

2. **Use Anonymity in Online Spaces:** When exploring breeding fantasies online, individuals should consider using pseudonyms or anonymous accounts. This practice can protect personal identities while allowing for engagement with like-minded individuals.

3. **Limit Digital Sharing:** Be cautious about sharing images, videos, or personal stories that could be linked back to one's real identity. Utilizing secure platforms with strong privacy settings can mitigate risks associated with digital sharing.

4. **Seek Private Spaces for Exploration:** Engaging in breeding fantasy in private settings, such as one's home or private retreats, can enhance the experience while maintaining confidentiality. This approach allows for intimacy without external pressures.

5. **Educate Partners on Privacy:** It is essential to communicate the importance of privacy to partners. Discussing the implications of sharing personal fantasies and experiences can foster mutual respect and understanding.

6. **Regularly Reassess Privacy Needs:** As relationships evolve, so do individual privacy needs. Regularly checking in with partners about comfort levels and boundaries can ensure that privacy concerns are continuously addressed.

Real-Life Examples

Consider a couple, Alex and Jamie, who are exploring breeding fantasies. Initially, they shared their experiences with a close friend, believing that this would enhance their intimacy. However, when the friend disclosed their private conversations to others, Alex and Jamie felt exposed and vulnerable. This incident prompted them to reassess their approach to privacy. They decided to limit discussions about their fantasies to only each other and established a rule to avoid sharing details with anyone outside their relationship.

Another example involves an individual, Taylor, who actively participates in online forums discussing breeding fantasies. Initially using their real name, Taylor faced unwanted attention and judgment from acquaintances who stumbled upon their posts. After this experience, Taylor created an anonymous profile, allowing them to engage with the community without fear of exposure. This change enabled Taylor to explore their desires openly while safeguarding their identity.

Conclusion

In conclusion, managing privacy concerns is a critical aspect of engaging in breeding fantasy and erotic pregnancy play. By understanding the importance of privacy, recognizing common concerns, and implementing effective strategies, individuals can create a safe and fulfilling environment for exploration. Ultimately, prioritizing privacy not only enhances the experience but also fosters trust and intimacy between partners. As the landscape of sexual exploration continues to evolve, maintaining a focus on privacy will ensure that individuals can navigate their desires with confidence and security.

Handling emotional triggers

In the realm of breeding fantasy and erotic pregnancy play, emotional triggers can arise unexpectedly, often linked to past experiences, societal pressures, or personal insecurities. Understanding and managing these triggers is essential for maintaining a safe and enjoyable experience for all participants involved. This section will explore the nature of emotional triggers, their potential impact on roleplay scenarios, and strategies for effectively addressing them.

Understanding Emotional Triggers

Emotional triggers are stimuli—whether they be words, actions, or situations—that evoke strong emotional responses based on past experiences. In the context of breeding fantasy, these triggers may relate to themes of fertility, motherhood, loss, or societal expectations around pregnancy. For instance, a participant may have a history of infertility or loss, making certain scenarios particularly sensitive.

The psychological framework surrounding emotional triggers can be understood through the lens of *Cognitive Behavioral Theory (CBT)*. CBT posits that our thoughts influence our feelings and behaviors. When a trigger is encountered, it can lead to a cascade of negative thoughts and emotions, which may disrupt the roleplay experience. For example, if a participant has a trigger related to the fear of abandonment, they may respond to a roleplay scenario involving separation with heightened anxiety or distress.

Identifying Personal Triggers

Before engaging in breeding fantasy roleplay, it is vital for participants to identify their emotional triggers. This process can involve self-reflection and open discussions with partners. Questions to consider include:

- What past experiences may influence my feelings about pregnancy or parenthood?
- Are there specific words or scenarios that evoke strong emotional reactions?
- How do I typically respond to feelings of discomfort or distress?

By acknowledging these triggers, participants can better prepare themselves for potential emotional responses during roleplay.

Communication and Negotiation

Effective communication is paramount in handling emotional triggers. Before engaging in breeding fantasy, partners should have an open dialogue about their boundaries, fears, and triggers. This can be facilitated through a negotiation process where each participant shares their comfort levels and establishes a safe space for exploration.

During this negotiation, it is beneficial to create a list of *safe words* or signals that can be used to pause or stop the roleplay if a trigger is encountered. For example, using the word "red" could signal an immediate halt to the scene, allowing participants to regroup and address any emotional distress.

Strategies for Managing Triggers

Once triggers are identified, participants can employ various strategies to manage them effectively:

- **Grounding Techniques:** These techniques help individuals remain present and connected to their bodies. Simple practices such as deep breathing, focusing on physical sensations, or engaging in mindfulness exercises can help mitigate the emotional impact of a trigger.

- **Pre-Roleplay Check-Ins:** Prior to beginning a scene, partners can engage in a check-in process to assess each other's emotional states. This can involve discussing any concerns or feelings that may have arisen since the last session, ensuring that both participants feel emotionally prepared for the roleplay.

- **Post-Roleplay Debriefing:** After a roleplay session, participants should take time to debrief their experiences. This can involve discussing what worked well, what felt uncomfortable, and how triggers were managed. This reflective practice fosters emotional intimacy and helps partners learn from each experience.

- **Therapeutic Support:** For individuals who find that emotional triggers significantly impact their ability to engage in breeding fantasy, seeking support from a therapist or counselor can be beneficial. A mental health professional can provide tools and strategies for coping with triggers and exploring underlying issues.

Examples of Emotional Triggers in Breeding Fantasy

To further illustrate the concept of emotional triggers, consider the following scenarios:

- **Scenario 1:** A participant who has experienced a miscarriage may find it difficult to engage in roleplay scenarios that involve pregnancy. The emotional weight of the past loss can surface unexpectedly, leading to feelings of sadness or anxiety. In this case, it is essential to establish clear boundaries around pregnancy-related themes and explore alternative scenarios that do not evoke painful memories.

- **Scenario 2:** Another participant may have a history of feeling judged for their desires surrounding breeding fantasies. In a roleplay scenario, they may become triggered by comments or actions that remind them of societal stigma. Open communication about these feelings can help partners navigate the scene with sensitivity and understanding, ensuring that the participant feels safe and accepted.

Conclusion

Handling emotional triggers in breeding fantasy requires a proactive approach centered on communication, self-awareness, and emotional support. By recognizing personal triggers, establishing clear boundaries, and employing strategies to manage emotional responses, participants can create a safe and fulfilling environment for exploring their desires. Ultimately, the key to navigating emotional triggers lies in fostering trust and intimacy between partners, allowing for deeper connections and more enriching experiences in the realm of erotic pregnancy play.

Roleplaying Scenarios

Natural conception

Natural conception is a deeply intimate and often exhilarating experience that many individuals and couples fantasize about. It involves the process of achieving pregnancy through unmediated sexual intercourse, where the male's sperm fertilizes the female's egg within her body. This section explores the dynamics of natural conception within the context of breeding fantasy, emphasizing the psychological, emotional, and physical aspects that enhance the allure of this scenario.

The Biological Process

At its core, natural conception hinges on a biological interplay between male and female reproductive systems. The female menstrual cycle plays a crucial role, typically lasting about 28 days, although variations are common. The cycle can be divided into several phases:

- **Menstrual Phase:** This phase marks the shedding of the uterine lining, lasting about 3 to 7 days.

- **Follicular Phase:** Following menstruation, the body prepares for ovulation, where follicles in the ovaries mature, and one egg is released.

- **Ovulation:** Approximately midway through the cycle, the mature egg is released from the ovary, making it available for fertilization. This is the peak time for conception.

- **Luteal Phase:** After ovulation, the body prepares for a potential pregnancy. If fertilization does not occur, the cycle restarts with menstruation.

The timing of intercourse relative to ovulation is critical. Engaging in sexual activity during the fertile window, which spans a few days before and after ovulation, maximizes the chances of conception. This knowledge can heighten the excitement and anticipation surrounding the act of trying to conceive.

Psychological Appeal of Natural Conception

The allure of natural conception within breeding fantasy is multifaceted. It often taps into deeply ingrained desires for connection, intimacy, and the creation of life. The act of conceiving can be perceived as a profound expression of love and commitment between partners. Moreover, the notion of surrendering to the primal instincts of reproduction can evoke feelings of vulnerability and trust.

$$\text{Fertility} = \frac{\text{Number of viable eggs} \times \text{Sperm count} \times \text{Sperm motility}}{\text{Cycle length}} \quad (2)$$

This equation illustrates that the likelihood of conception is influenced by various factors, including the quality of the sperm and eggs, as well as the timing within the menstrual cycle. The thrill of trying to conceive can be amplified by the anticipation of potential pregnancy, transforming the act of intercourse into a shared goal.

Roleplaying Natural Conception

In the context of erotic roleplay, natural conception scenarios can be creatively explored. Couples might engage in roleplaying that emphasizes the excitement and spontaneity of trying to conceive. Here are a few ideas for roleplaying natural conception:

- **The Fertile Weekend:** Plan a weekend getaway during the peak of the fertile window. Create an atmosphere of intimacy and relaxation, allowing the couple to focus on each other and the possibility of conception.

- **The Surprise:** One partner could surprise the other with a romantic evening, emphasizing the intention to conceive. This could involve romantic gestures, such as candles, soft music, and intimate conversations about their desires for a family.

- **The Ritual:** Establish a pre-conception ritual that both partners participate in, which could include affirmations, setting intentions, or even lighthearted discussions about potential baby names.

These scenarios not only enhance intimacy but also encourage open communication about desires, fears, and expectations regarding conception.

Challenges and Considerations

While the fantasy of natural conception can be thrilling, it is essential to acknowledge the potential challenges that may arise. These include:

- **Fertility Issues:** Couples may face difficulties conceiving due to various factors, including age, medical conditions, or lifestyle choices. It's crucial to approach these topics with sensitivity and understanding.

- **Emotional Stress:** The pressure to conceive can lead to anxiety and frustration. Open communication about feelings and expectations can help mitigate these stresses.

- **Societal Pressures:** Societal expectations surrounding family planning can create additional stress. Couples should focus on their desires rather than external judgments.

Incorporating discussions about these challenges into roleplay can foster deeper emotional connections and enhance the experience of trying to conceive.

Conclusion

Natural conception is a complex interplay of biology, psychology, and emotion, making it a rich theme for exploration within breeding fantasy. By understanding the biological processes involved, embracing the psychological appeal, and navigating the challenges, couples can create a fulfilling and intimate experience. Roleplaying scenarios centered around natural conception can deepen connections and foster a shared sense of purpose, ultimately enhancing the eroticism and intimacy of the experience. The journey toward conception, while fraught with potential difficulties, can also be a profoundly rewarding adventure that strengthens the bond between partners.

Exploring fertility and ovulation

Fertility and ovulation are central to the breeding fantasy, serving as the biological foundation upon which many erotic scenarios are built. Understanding these concepts not only enhances the roleplay experience but also allows participants to engage with the underlying themes of desire, power, and intimacy.

The Science of Fertility

Fertility is defined as the natural capability to produce offspring. In humans, this is primarily influenced by a variety of physiological factors, including hormonal levels, reproductive health, and age. The menstrual cycle, which typically lasts 28 days, is pivotal in determining a woman's fertility window.

The cycle can be divided into several phases:

- **Menstrual Phase:** Days 1-5, when menstruation occurs.

- **Follicular Phase:** Days 1-13, during which follicles in the ovaries mature.

- **Ovulation:** Around day 14, when a mature egg is released from the ovary.

- **Luteal Phase:** Days 15-28, where the body prepares for a potential pregnancy.

The key event in this cycle is ovulation, where the luteinizing hormone (LH) surges, triggering the release of an egg. The timing of ovulation is crucial for conception, as the egg remains viable for approximately 12-24 hours post-ovulation, while sperm can survive in the female reproductive tract for up to five days.

Fertility Awareness Methods

Fertility Awareness Methods (FAM) are techniques used to predict ovulation and identify fertile windows. These methods can be particularly useful in the context of breeding fantasy roleplay. Some popular FAM include:

- **Basal Body Temperature (BBT) Charting:** Tracking body temperature daily to identify the slight increase that occurs after ovulation.

- **Cervical Mucus Monitoring:** Observing changes in cervical mucus consistency, which becomes clear and stretchy during ovulation.

- **Calendar Method:** Keeping a record of menstrual cycles to predict future ovulation.

The integration of these methods into roleplay scenarios can heighten the sense of anticipation and excitement around conception. For example, a couple may roleplay the act of checking for ovulation signs, heightening the emotional stakes of their encounter.

Common Challenges in Fertility

While the biological aspects of fertility are fascinating, they can also present challenges. Issues such as irregular cycles, hormonal imbalances, and reproductive health conditions (e.g., Polycystic Ovary Syndrome (PCOS), endometriosis) can complicate the process of conception.

In roleplay, these challenges can be incorporated to explore deeper emotional narratives. For instance, a couple may roleplay the frustration and longing associated with trying to conceive amidst these obstacles. This can lead to rich storytelling opportunities, allowing participants to express vulnerability and intimacy.

The Emotional Landscape of Fertility

Fertility is not merely a biological process; it is deeply intertwined with emotions and personal identity. The desire to conceive can evoke a spectrum of feelings ranging from hope and joy to anxiety and despair.

In the context of breeding fantasy, exploring these emotions can enhance the realism and depth of roleplay. For example, a scenario may involve one partner expressing their fears about not being able to conceive, while the other offers reassurance and support. This dynamic can create a powerful bond, reinforcing the intimacy of the experience.

Roleplaying Fertility and Ovulation

When incorporating fertility and ovulation into breeding fantasy roleplay, consider the following scenarios:

- **The Countdown to Ovulation:** Engage in a playful countdown to ovulation, where partners express excitement and anticipation through intimate acts leading up to the fertile window.

- **Fertility Rituals:** Create personalized rituals that celebrate the act of trying to conceive, such as special dates or settings that hold significance for the couple.

- **Medical Play:** Explore the themes of fertility through medical roleplay, where one partner takes on the role of a fertility specialist guiding the other through the process of conception.

By creatively integrating these elements, participants can deepen their connection while exploring the nuances of fertility and ovulation in a safe and consensual environment.

Conclusion

Exploring fertility and ovulation within the context of breeding fantasy opens up a rich tapestry of emotional and physical experiences. By understanding the science behind these concepts and incorporating them into roleplay scenarios, participants can enhance their intimacy and connection, creating a fulfilling and pleasurable experience. The key lies in open communication, consent, and a willingness to explore the depths of desire together.

The excitement of trying to conceive

The journey of trying to conceive can be an exhilarating and deeply intimate experience for couples exploring breeding fantasies. This phase is often characterized by a blend of anticipation, hope, and a sense of shared purpose. Understanding the psychological and emotional dynamics at play during this period can enhance the roleplay experience and deepen the connection between partners.

Psychological Dynamics

The excitement of trying to conceive can be understood through several psychological lenses. The anticipation of potential pregnancy can evoke feelings of joy and excitement, as well as anxiety and fear. This duality is rooted in the significant life changes that pregnancy entails, both desired and feared. For many, the act of trying to conceive becomes a ritual filled with hope, intimacy, and a sense of unity.

Anticipation and Desire The anticipation of conception often heightens desire, making intimacy more thrilling. The idea of creating life can transform sexual encounters into sacred acts, where every touch and kiss is imbued with meaning. This can lead to a heightened state of arousal, as partners engage in a dance of seduction that is both playful and serious. Roleplaying scenarios can enhance this experience by incorporating elements that emphasize the thrill of the chase, such as:

- Setting the scene with romantic lighting and music.
- Engaging in playful banter about the future family.
- Incorporating fertility symbols, such as fruits or flowers, to represent growth and potential.

Methods of Roleplaying Natural Conception

Roleplaying natural conception can involve various techniques that simulate the experience. Here are some methods to enhance the excitement:

Fertility Awareness Understanding the menstrual cycle and the timing of ovulation can add a layer of realism to the roleplay. Couples can engage in discussions about fertility signs, such as basal body temperature and cervical mucus changes. This knowledge can be woven into the narrative, creating a sense of urgency and excitement about the fertile window.

Playful Challenges Incorporating playful challenges can amplify the thrill. For instance, partners might create a game where they must engage in specific acts of intimacy leading up to ovulation, turning the act of trying to conceive into a fun and engaging competition. This can include:

- Setting specific "conception dates" that are treated like special occasions.
- Creating a countdown to ovulation, building anticipation for intimacy.
- Rewarding each other for participation with small tokens of affection or surprises.

Exploring Emotional Connections

The act of trying to conceive can also evoke a range of emotions that can be explored during roleplay. Partners might discuss their feelings about parenthood, their hopes for the future, and any fears they may have. This emotional exploration can strengthen the bond between partners and create a safe space for vulnerability.

Addressing Fears and Insecurities While the excitement of trying to conceive is palpable, it is essential to acknowledge the fears and insecurities that may arise. Concerns about fertility, the health of a potential pregnancy, and the responsibilities of parenthood can weigh heavily on couples. Roleplaying can provide an opportunity to address these fears in a supportive environment. For example, partners can:

- Share their worries about pregnancy and parenting, allowing for open communication.
- Roleplay scenarios where they reassure each other, reinforcing their commitment and support.
- Create a safe word or signal to pause the roleplay if emotions become overwhelming.

Incorporating Rituals and Traditions

Rituals can enhance the excitement of trying to conceive by creating a sense of significance around the experience. Couples might consider incorporating traditions from their cultural backgrounds or inventing their own. These rituals can serve as a powerful reminder of the shared journey they are on, such as:

- Lighting candles or setting up an altar dedicated to fertility.
- Writing down their hopes and dreams for their future family and sharing them with each other.

- Celebrating each month of trying with a special date night or intimate gathering.

Conclusion

The excitement of trying to conceive is a rich tapestry of emotions, desires, and intimate connections. By embracing the psychological dynamics at play and incorporating roleplaying techniques, couples can enhance their experiences and deepen their bond. As they navigate this journey together, the thrill of potential parenthood can transform into a powerful catalyst for intimacy, trust, and love.

Methods of roleplaying natural conception

Roleplaying natural conception can be a deeply intimate and thrilling experience for partners who wish to explore the dynamics of fertility, desire, and the potential for new life. This section delves into various methods and techniques to effectively roleplay natural conception scenarios while prioritizing consent, communication, and emotional safety.

Understanding the Context

Before engaging in roleplay, it is crucial to establish a shared understanding of what natural conception entails. This includes recognizing the biological processes involved, such as ovulation and fertilization, as well as the emotional and psychological aspects that accompany the desire to conceive. Partners should have open discussions about their motivations for engaging in this fantasy, ensuring they are both on the same page regarding boundaries and expectations.

Methods of Roleplaying Natural Conception

1. **Setting the Scene** Creating an appropriate environment can enhance the roleplaying experience. Consider the following elements:

    - **Location:** Choose a private and comfortable space where both partners feel safe. This could be a bedroom, a secluded outdoor area, or even a designated playroom.

    - **Props:** Utilize props that enhance the realism of the scenario. This could include items like fertility calendars, ovulation tests, or even romantic decorations that set the mood.

ROLEPLAYING SCENARIOS 57

- **Costumes:** Dressing in a way that reflects the characters you are embodying can add depth to the roleplay. For instance, one partner may dress as a doctor or a fertility specialist, while the other may take on the role of a hopeful parent.

2. **Exploring Fertility Awareness** Understanding and incorporating fertility awareness into the roleplay can heighten the experience. Partners can engage in activities such as:

- **Tracking Ovulation:** Roleplay the process of tracking ovulation through calendars or apps. Discussing the signs of fertility, such as changes in cervical mucus or basal body temperature, can add an educational element to the fantasy.

- **Fertility Rituals:** Create rituals that symbolize the desire to conceive. This could involve lighting candles, meditating, or performing a special dance that signifies the union of energies.

3. **Engaging in Intimate Conversations** Intimacy is a vital component of natural conception roleplay. Engage in conversations that reflect the desires, hopes, and fears surrounding conception. Examples include:

- **Discussing Future Dreams:** Share fantasies about what it would be like to become parents. Discuss names, parenting styles, and the kind of family you envision.

- **Expressing Vulnerabilities:** Open up about any fears or anxieties related to conception. This could involve discussing past experiences, societal pressures, or personal insecurities.

4. **Physical Connection** The physical aspect of roleplaying natural conception is crucial. Consider the following methods:

- **Foreplay:** Engage in extended foreplay that emphasizes intimacy and connection. This could include sensual massages, kissing, and exploring each other's bodies.

- **Simulated Intercourse:** Roleplay the act of conception through simulated intercourse. This can involve discussing the process, using language that reflects the desire to conceive, and focusing on the emotional connection during the act.

+ **Incorporating Fertility Tools:** Use props like fertility lubricants or supplements that enhance the experience. Discuss how these tools play a role in the conception process.

5. **Incorporating Aftercare** Aftercare is essential in any roleplay scenario, especially one that involves deep emotional themes like conception. Aftercare can include:

+ **Cuddling and Affection:** Spend time in close physical proximity, providing comfort and reassurance after the intensity of the roleplay.

+ **Debriefing:** Have a conversation about the experience. Discuss what felt good, any discomforts, and how both partners can improve future roleplay sessions.

+ **Emotional Check-ins:** Ensure both partners feel emotionally safe and validated. Address any feelings that may have arisen during the roleplay.

Potential Challenges and Solutions

While roleplaying natural conception can be fulfilling, it may also present challenges. Here are common issues and potential solutions:

1. **Emotional Triggers** The topic of conception can evoke strong emotions. It is essential to:

+ **Identify Triggers:** Before engaging in roleplay, discuss any potential emotional triggers. This could include past experiences with fertility struggles or societal pressures.

+ **Establish Safewords:** Create a system for halting the roleplay if it becomes overwhelming. Safewords should be clear and respected by both partners.

2. **Miscommunication** Clear communication is vital to avoid misunderstandings. To enhance communication:

+ **Pre-Roleplay Discussions:** Have thorough discussions before engaging in roleplay. Outline boundaries, desires, and expectations to ensure both partners are aligned.

+ **Active Listening:** During the roleplay, practice active listening. Pay attention to verbal and non-verbal cues to gauge comfort levels.

3. **Societal Judgment** Engaging in breeding fantasies may lead to societal judgment. To navigate this:

- **Creating a Safe Space:** Ensure that the roleplay occurs in a private setting where external judgment is minimized.
- **Educating Partners:** If discussing the fantasy with others, be prepared to educate them about the consensual nature of the roleplay and the importance of personal exploration.

Conclusion

Roleplaying natural conception offers a unique opportunity for partners to explore their desires, deepen their emotional connection, and engage in a fantasy that intertwines intimacy with the complexities of fertility. By establishing a safe and consensual environment, partners can navigate the nuances of this roleplay, ensuring that both individuals feel empowered and fulfilled in their exploration. Embracing the journey of natural conception roleplay can lead to profound insights, enhanced intimacy, and a deeper understanding of each other's desires and boundaries.

Exploring Reproductive Health and Issues

Reproductive health is a critical aspect of human sexuality, encompassing a wide range of physical, emotional, and social factors that affect individuals' ability to reproduce and maintain a healthy sexual life. In the context of breeding fantasies and erotic pregnancy play, understanding reproductive health issues is essential to ensure that all participants engage in safe, consensual, and informed practices. This section will explore common reproductive health issues, their implications for roleplay scenarios, and how to navigate these topics within the framework of erotic fantasies.

Understanding Reproductive Health

Reproductive health is defined by the World Health Organization (WHO) as a state of complete physical, mental, and social well-being in all matters relating to the reproductive system. It involves the ability to have a satisfying and safe sex life, the capability to reproduce, and the freedom to decide if, when, and how often to do so. This definition highlights the importance of education, access to healthcare, and the removal of stigma surrounding reproductive issues.

Common Reproductive Health Issues

Several reproductive health issues can impact individuals engaged in breeding fantasies. Understanding these issues is vital for ensuring that fantasies remain safe and enjoyable. Below are some common reproductive health concerns:

- **Infertility:** Infertility is defined as the inability to conceive after one year of unprotected intercourse. This can be due to various factors, including hormonal imbalances, anatomical issues, or lifestyle factors. In roleplay scenarios, infertility can be a sensitive topic, and partners should approach it with care and understanding.

- **Sexually Transmitted Infections (STIs):** STIs can pose serious risks to reproductive health and can complicate pregnancy. Engaging in safe sex practices, such as using condoms, is crucial to prevent the transmission of STIs. In breeding fantasies, partners may want to incorporate discussions about STI testing and prevention into their roleplay.

- **Pregnancy Complications:** Complications such as gestational diabetes, preeclampsia, and ectopic pregnancies can arise during pregnancy. These issues can be incorporated into roleplay scenarios, but it is essential to approach them with sensitivity and awareness of their emotional impact.

- **Menstrual Disorders:** Conditions such as polycystic ovary syndrome (PCOS) or endometriosis can affect fertility and overall reproductive health. Understanding these disorders can help partners navigate their fantasies and address any concerns that may arise during roleplay.

- **Mental Health:** Mental health plays a significant role in reproductive health. Issues such as anxiety, depression, or trauma can affect individuals' desire to engage in sexual activities or fantasies. It is essential to create a safe space for partners to discuss their mental health and how it may influence their roleplay experiences.

The Role of Education and Communication

Education about reproductive health is crucial for individuals engaging in breeding fantasies. Partners should feel empowered to discuss their reproductive health history, any existing conditions, and their comfort levels with various aspects of roleplay. Open communication fosters trust and allows partners to establish boundaries that respect each other's health and well-being.

Incorporating Reproductive Health Issues into Roleplay

When exploring breeding fantasies, it is essential to consider how reproductive health issues can be integrated into roleplay scenarios. Here are some examples of how to approach this:

- **Infertility Roleplay:** Partners may choose to roleplay a scenario where they are trying to conceive but face challenges due to infertility. This can open up discussions about emotional support, the importance of communication, and exploring alternative methods of conception, such as artificial insemination.

- **STI Awareness:** Roleplaying scenarios can include discussions about STI testing and safe sex practices. This can enhance the realism of the fantasy while emphasizing the importance of health and safety.

- **Pregnancy Complications:** Partners may choose to explore scenarios involving pregnancy complications, allowing them to navigate the emotional and physical challenges that may arise. This can lead to deeper intimacy and understanding of each other's fears and desires.

- **Menstrual Disorders:** Incorporating the realities of menstrual disorders into roleplay can create a more authentic experience. This can involve discussions about how these conditions affect sexual desire and reproductive choices.

Navigating Emotional Responses

Engaging in breeding fantasies can evoke a wide range of emotions, especially when reproductive health issues are involved. Partners should be prepared to navigate these emotional responses through:

- **Check-ins:** Regularly checking in with each other during roleplay can help partners gauge comfort levels and address any emotional triggers that may arise.

- **Aftercare:** Providing aftercare following roleplay is essential for emotional well-being. This can include cuddling, discussing feelings, and ensuring that both partners feel safe and supported.

- **Therapeutic Support:** If partners experience significant emotional distress, seeking support from a therapist or counselor specializing in sexual health can be beneficial. This can help individuals process their feelings and enhance their overall experience.

Conclusion

Exploring reproductive health and issues within the context of breeding fantasies is essential for creating safe, consensual, and fulfilling experiences. By understanding common reproductive health concerns, fostering open communication, and navigating emotional responses, partners can deepen their connection and enhance their roleplay. Ultimately, prioritizing reproductive health not only enriches the fantasy but also promotes a healthier, more satisfying sexual relationship.

Roleplaying during the fertile window

The fertile window is a critical concept in both reproductive health and breeding fantasy. It represents the period during a woman's menstrual cycle when she is most likely to conceive. Understanding this window not only enhances the realism of roleplaying scenarios but also deepens the psychological engagement for participants.

Understanding the Fertile Window

The fertile window typically spans about six days: the five days leading up to ovulation and the day of ovulation itself. This period is crucial for couples trying to conceive, as the chances of pregnancy are highest during this time. The physiological changes that occur during this window can be fascinating to explore in roleplay.

$$\text{Fertile Window} = \text{Ovulation Day} - 5 \text{ to Ovulation Day} \qquad (3)$$

In roleplaying scenarios, this can translate into heightened emotions, increased intimacy, and a sense of urgency. Participants may feel a mix of excitement and anxiety, which can enhance the eroticism of the scene.

Setting the Scene for Roleplay

To effectively roleplay during the fertile window, it is essential to set the stage. This can include:

- **Creating a Realistic Environment**: Use props and settings that evoke the feeling of intimacy and urgency associated with the fertile window. Dim lighting, soft fabrics, and romantic music can enhance the mood.

- **Incorporating Timing**: Roleplay can be timed to align with the actual ovulation cycle. For instance, using an ovulation tracker or apps can add an element of authenticity.

- **Emotional Engagement**: Discuss the feelings and desires associated with trying to conceive. This can lead to deeper emotional connections and a more immersive experience.

Roleplaying Scenarios

Several scenarios can be explored during the fertile window:

The Excitement of Trying to Conceive This scenario focuses on the thrill and anticipation of conception. Participants can roleplay as a couple who are actively trying to conceive, discussing their hopes, fears, and desires. This can involve playful banter about the timing, intimate moments that lead to conception, and expressions of joy or anxiety about the outcome.

Natural Conception Roleplay In this scenario, participants can reenact the act of natural conception, emphasizing the physical and emotional aspects. This includes foreplay, intimacy, and the culmination of their efforts. The excitement can be amplified by incorporating elements of spontaneity and urgency, reflecting the real-life pressures associated with conception.

Exploring Fertility and Ovulation Roleplaying can include educational elements about fertility and ovulation. Participants can take on roles such as a doctor and patient, where they discuss reproductive health, fertility issues, or even explore the idea of fertility treatments. This adds depth to the fantasy while maintaining a focus on the fertile window.

Intimacy During the Fertile Window This scenario emphasizes the emotional connection and intimacy that can occur during this time. It can involve slow, sensual interactions that highlight the bond between partners. Discussing fantasies about family, future children, and shared dreams can enhance the emotional engagement.

Communication and Consent

As with all roleplay scenarios, communication and consent are paramount. Participants should discuss their boundaries, desires, and any potential triggers related to fertility and conception. Establishing safewords and check-ins during the roleplay can ensure that both partners feel safe and respected throughout the experience.

Challenges and Considerations

While roleplaying during the fertile window can be exhilarating, it can also present challenges:

- **Emotional Triggers**: Discussions or roleplays around fertility can evoke strong emotions. Participants should be aware of any past experiences related to pregnancy or conception that may surface during the roleplay.

- **Societal Stigma**: Engaging in breeding fantasies can sometimes attract societal judgment. Participants should be prepared to navigate these feelings and support each other in maintaining a positive mindset.

- **Balancing Fantasy and Reality**: It is crucial to maintain a distinction between fantasy and real-life desires. Participants should regularly check in with each other to ensure that the roleplay remains enjoyable and consensual.

Aftercare and Reflection

Aftercare is an essential component of any roleplay, especially one that involves emotional themes like fertility. Participants should take time to reconnect after the roleplay, discussing their feelings, experiences, and any emotional responses that arose during the scenario. This can help solidify the bond between partners and ensure a positive experience.

In conclusion, roleplaying during the fertile window can be a deeply enriching experience, blending eroticism with emotional intimacy. By understanding the physiological aspects, setting the scene, and maintaining open communication, participants can explore this fantasy in a safe and consensual manner, enhancing their connection and deepening their understanding of each other's desires.

Intimacy during pregnancy

Intimacy during pregnancy encompasses a complex interplay of emotional, physical, and psychological factors that can significantly enhance or challenge the relationship between partners. As the body undergoes profound transformations, both partners may experience shifts in their desires, needs, and perceptions of intimacy. This section explores the dynamics of intimacy during pregnancy, addressing common challenges, theoretical perspectives, and practical examples to help couples navigate this unique phase of their relationship.

The Emotional Landscape

Pregnancy can evoke a wide array of emotions, ranging from joy and excitement to anxiety and insecurity. The expectant partner may grapple with body image issues, hormonal fluctuations, and the anticipation of motherhood, all of which can impact their desire for intimacy. The non-pregnant partner may also experience feelings of helplessness or confusion about how to support their partner while maintaining their own needs for connection.

Theoretical Perspectives   From a psychological standpoint, attachment theory provides valuable insights into how couples navigate intimacy during pregnancy. According to Bowlby's attachment theory, the emotional bond formed between partners can influence their ability to communicate needs and seek comfort. A secure attachment style fosters open communication and emotional support, while insecure attachment may lead to misunderstandings and emotional withdrawal.

Moreover, the concept of *relational intimacy* is crucial in understanding how couples can maintain closeness during this transformative period. Relational intimacy involves the sharing of thoughts, feelings, and experiences, fostering a sense of connection that transcends physical interactions. As partners navigate the challenges of pregnancy, prioritizing emotional intimacy can help strengthen their bond.

Physical Changes and Challenges

The physical changes that accompany pregnancy can pose challenges to intimacy. The expectant partner may experience discomfort, fatigue, and body image concerns, which can diminish their interest in sexual activity. It is essential for both partners to communicate openly about their physical needs and limitations during this time.

Common Issues

- **Body Image Concerns:** Many pregnant individuals struggle with body image as their bodies change. It is vital for partners to engage in affirming conversations that celebrate the beauty of pregnancy and reinforce feelings of desirability.

- **Physical Discomfort:** Pregnancy can bring about various physical discomforts, such as back pain, nausea, and fatigue. Partners should explore alternative forms of intimacy, such as cuddling, massage, and non-sexual physical touch, to maintain connection without the pressure of sexual activity.

- **Hormonal Fluctuations:** Hormonal changes can affect libido and mood. Open discussions about these changes can help partners navigate their evolving sexual dynamics.

Strategies for Enhancing Intimacy

To foster intimacy during pregnancy, couples can adopt several strategies that prioritize emotional connection and physical comfort.

1. **Open Communication** Establishing a safe space for open dialogue about desires, fears, and expectations is crucial. Partners should regularly check in with each other, discussing what feels good and what does not. This ongoing conversation can help mitigate misunderstandings and reinforce emotional intimacy.

2. **Exploring Non-Sexual Intimacy** Non-sexual forms of intimacy can be incredibly fulfilling during pregnancy. Activities such as cuddling, kissing, and intimate conversations can nurture the emotional bond without the pressure of sexual performance. Additionally, exploring activities like joint prenatal yoga or attending birthing classes together can enhance connection and foster shared experiences.

3. **Embracing the Changes Together** Couples can engage in activities that celebrate the pregnancy journey, such as creating a pregnancy journal, taking maternity photos, or attending prenatal appointments together. These shared experiences can deepen emotional intimacy and provide opportunities for partners to express their feelings and support each other.

4. **Seeking Professional Guidance** If intimacy challenges persist, seeking the guidance of a therapist or counselor specializing in relationships can provide valuable tools and insights. Professional support can facilitate constructive conversations and help couples navigate any underlying issues that may be affecting their intimacy.

Case Studies and Examples

Consider the case of Jamie and Alex, a couple navigating Jamie's pregnancy. Initially, Jamie felt self-conscious about her changing body, leading to a decrease in her interest in sexual intimacy. Alex, recognizing the shift, initiated conversations about their feelings and explored alternative forms of intimacy, such as long walks and shared baths. By prioritizing emotional connection and affirming Jamie's beauty, they were able to maintain a strong bond throughout the pregnancy.

In another example, Maya and Sam found that attending prenatal classes together not only provided them with valuable information but also fostered a sense of teamwork and shared purpose. They embraced the opportunity to connect with other expectant couples, which helped normalize their experiences and reinforced their emotional intimacy.

Conclusion

Intimacy during pregnancy is a multifaceted experience that requires patience, understanding, and open communication. By acknowledging the emotional and physical changes that accompany this journey, couples can cultivate a deeper connection that transcends traditional notions of intimacy. Emphasizing emotional support, exploring alternative forms of closeness, and engaging in shared experiences can help partners navigate the complexities of intimacy during pregnancy, ultimately strengthening their bond as they prepare for parenthood together.

Fantasizing about labor and birth

Fantasizing about labor and birth can evoke a complex tapestry of emotions and desires, intertwining the themes of creation, vulnerability, and power dynamics. For many, the act of roleplaying labor and birth scenarios serves as a profound exploration of the physical and emotional landscapes associated with pregnancy, while also tapping into the primal instincts of reproduction.

Theoretical Framework

The psychological underpinnings of labor and birth fantasies can be analyzed through various lenses, including psychoanalytic theory, which posits that such fantasies may arise from deep-seated desires for nurturing, control, and transformation. Sigmund Freud's theories on the unconscious mind suggest that fantasies about childbirth may symbolize the desire for new beginnings and the manifestation of one's creative potential.

Moreover, the concept of *eroticized birth* posits that the physiological processes of labor can be intertwined with sexual arousal. This perspective aligns with the work of researchers such as Dr. Jessica D. H. McLain, who emphasizes the interplay between sexuality and reproduction in her studies on maternal sexuality. The idea that labor can be seen as an erotic experience challenges conventional narratives surrounding childbirth, inviting individuals to reclaim the experience as one of empowerment and sensuality.

Common Themes in Labor and Birth Fantasies

1. **Power Dynamics**: Fantasies surrounding labor often explore themes of power exchange. The submissive role may be characterized by surrendering to the natural process of birth, while the dominant partner may take on the role of a supportive figure, guiding the experience. This dynamic can enhance feelings of safety and trust, allowing for a deeper exploration of vulnerability.

2. **Physical Sensation**: Many individuals fantasize about the intense physical sensations associated with labor. The rhythmic contractions and the culmination of effort can evoke feelings of euphoria and accomplishment. This focus on physicality can heighten arousal, as the body becomes a site of both pleasure and pain.

3. **Intimacy and Connection**: Labor and birth fantasies often emphasize the intimate connection between partners. The shared experience of labor can serve to deepen emotional bonds, fostering a sense of unity and collaboration. This intimacy can be enhanced through roleplay scenarios that prioritize communication and mutual support.

4. **Ritual and Ceremony**: The act of giving birth can be framed as a ritualistic experience, with specific practices and symbols that enhance the fantasy. Incorporating elements such as candles, music, or specific clothing can create a sacred space for the roleplay, enhancing the emotional and psychological impact of the experience.

Examples of Roleplay Scenarios

1. **The Home Birth**: In this scenario, the couple creates a safe and intimate environment, simulating a home birth. The submissive partner may roleplay as the laboring individual, expressing sensations and emotions while the dominant partner

provides support. This can include physical assistance, such as massage or guiding breathing techniques, enhancing the sense of connection and safety.

2. **The Medical Setting**: This scenario introduces the dynamics of a hospital birth, with the dominant partner taking on the role of a medical professional or supportive partner. The submissive partner may experience the sensations of labor while navigating the clinical environment. This can include the use of props such as medical instruments or hospital gowns, heightening the realism of the roleplay.

3. **Fantasy Labor**: In this imaginative scenario, the partners explore a fantastical version of labor, incorporating elements of magic or mythology. The submissive partner may roleplay as a mythical creature giving birth, while the dominant partner acts as a guardian or protector. This allows for a creative exploration of the themes of birth and creation in a non-traditional context.

Challenges and Considerations

While fantasizing about labor and birth can be a fulfilling exploration of intimacy and desire, it is essential to approach these scenarios with care and consideration.

1. **Emotional Triggers**: For some, the themes of labor and birth may evoke strong emotional responses, particularly if there are past traumas or unresolved feelings associated with childbirth. It is crucial to establish clear communication and consent, ensuring that both partners are comfortable engaging in these fantasies.

2. **Physical Safety**: Roleplaying labor should prioritize physical safety. Partners should agree on boundaries and establish safewords to ensure that both individuals can navigate the experience without discomfort or harm.

3. **Aftercare**: The intensity of labor and birth roleplay may necessitate thorough aftercare, as both partners may experience a range of emotions post-experience. Engaging in supportive practices, such as cuddling or discussing feelings, can help both partners process the experience and reinforce emotional bonds.

Conclusion

Fantasizing about labor and birth offers a rich landscape for exploration, allowing individuals to engage with their desires, fears, and fantasies surrounding reproduction. By navigating the complexities of power dynamics, physical sensations, and emotional intimacy, partners can create a unique and fulfilling experience that transcends traditional narratives of childbirth. Through careful communication, consent, and aftercare, labor and birth roleplay can become a profound journey of connection and self-discovery, celebrating the intricate interplay of sexuality and reproduction.

Postpartum roleplay and recovery

Postpartum roleplay and recovery is an often-overlooked aspect of breeding fantasy that can provide a rich and nuanced exploration of intimacy, vulnerability, and the physical and emotional changes that follow childbirth. This section delves into the dynamics of postpartum roleplay, addressing both the theoretical underpinnings and practical considerations for those who wish to incorporate this element into their erotic experiences.

Understanding Postpartum Roleplay

Postpartum roleplay allows individuals to engage with the complex realities of the post-birth experience, including themes of nurturing, healing, and the transformation of identity. This form of roleplay can serve as a powerful tool for exploring the following:

- **Emotional Vulnerability:** The postpartum period is often marked by a significant emotional shift. Roleplaying can create a safe space to explore feelings of joy, anxiety, and even postpartum depression in a controlled environment.

- **Physical Changes:** Participants can embody the physical changes that occur after childbirth, such as body image issues and the healing process. This can be a way to confront and embrace these changes through fantasy.

- **Nurturing Dynamics:** Postpartum roleplay often emphasizes caregiving roles, allowing participants to explore dynamics of nurturing, support, and dependency.

Theoretical Framework

The psychological appeal of postpartum roleplay can be understood through the lens of several theories:

- **Attachment Theory:** This theory posits that early experiences with caregivers shape emotional bonds throughout life. Postpartum roleplay can mimic these dynamics, allowing participants to explore attachment styles and their impacts on relationships.

- **Embodiment Theory:** This theory suggests that our bodily experiences influence our perceptions and emotions. Engaging in postpartum roleplay allows participants to reconnect with their bodies in a new way, fostering a sense of agency and empowerment.

- **Feminist Theory:** Feminist perspectives can provide insights into the societal pressures surrounding motherhood and femininity. Postpartum roleplay can challenge traditional narratives and empower participants to reclaim their narratives.

Practical Considerations

When engaging in postpartum roleplay, it is crucial to establish clear communication and consent to ensure a positive experience. Here are some practical considerations:

- **Setting Boundaries:** Discuss the specific aspects of postpartum experiences that participants are comfortable exploring. This can include physical sensations, emotional states, and particular scenarios.

- **Emotional Check-ins:** Regularly check in with each other during the roleplay to assess comfort levels and emotional responses. This can help mitigate any unexpected triggers.

- **Aftercare:** Aftercare is essential in postpartum roleplay to address any emotional fallout and reinforce the bond between participants. This can include cuddling, verbal affirmations, or other comforting activities.

Roleplay Scenarios

Here are some examples of postpartum roleplay scenarios that can enhance the experience:

- **Nurturing the Newborn:** One partner can take on the role of a caregiver, tending to a "newborn" (which can be a doll or plush toy), while the other partner embodies the postpartum individual. This scenario can highlight themes of nurturing and support.

- **Healing Conversations:** Roleplay intimate conversations about the challenges of recovery, including physical discomfort, emotional struggles, and the joys of motherhood. This can foster deeper emotional connections.

- **Body Exploration:** Engage in a roleplay that focuses on body exploration, allowing the postpartum individual to express feelings about their body and receive affirmations from their partner.

Challenges and Considerations

While postpartum roleplay can be fulfilling, it also presents unique challenges:

- **Emotional Triggers:** Participants may encounter unexpected emotional triggers related to their own experiences with childbirth or postpartum recovery. It is essential to remain sensitive to these reactions and adapt the roleplay accordingly.

- **Societal Stigma:** Engaging in postpartum roleplay may evoke societal judgments or stigma surrounding motherhood and sexuality. Participants should prepare to discuss these concerns and support each other.

- **Balancing Fantasy and Reality:** It is crucial to maintain a clear distinction between roleplay and real-life experiences. Participants should regularly communicate to ensure that fantasies do not overshadow the realities of parenting and recovery.

Conclusion

Postpartum roleplay and recovery can serve as a powerful means of exploring the complexities of parenthood, intimacy, and personal transformation. By engaging in this form of roleplay, individuals can foster deeper connections with their partners, confront societal taboos, and embrace the multifaceted nature of their identities. As with all forms of erotic roleplay, the key lies in open communication, consent, and a commitment to mutual support and understanding.

Artificial insemination

Artificial insemination (AI) is a medical procedure that involves the deliberate introduction of sperm into a female's reproductive system for the purpose of achieving pregnancy without sexual intercourse. This method has gained popularity not only for its medical applications but also as a theme in erotic roleplay, particularly within the context of breeding fantasies. In this section, we will explore the various aspects of artificial insemination, including its techniques, psychological implications, and the integration of this theme into erotic roleplay scenarios.

Understanding the Process of Artificial Insemination

Artificial insemination can be performed using different techniques, primarily categorized into two types: intrauterine insemination (IUI) and intracervical insemination (ICI).

- **Intrauterine Insemination (IUI):** This method involves placing sperm directly into the uterus using a thin catheter. This technique is often preferred due to its higher success rates compared to ICI, as it bypasses the cervix and allows sperm to be deposited closer to the egg.

- **Intracervical Insemination (ICI):** This method involves placing sperm into the cervical canal. While it is less invasive than IUI, it may be less effective as the sperm must travel through the cervix to reach the uterus.

The choice of technique often depends on various factors, including the couple's fertility issues, the quality of the sperm, and the timing of ovulation.

Roleplaying Insemination Techniques

Incorporating artificial insemination into erotic roleplay can add layers of complexity and excitement. Here are some scenarios that can be explored:

- **The Medical Setting:** Roleplay can take place in a clinical environment, where one partner assumes the role of a medical professional. This scenario can involve discussions about fertility, procedures, and the emotional aspects of insemination. The sterile environment can heighten the sense of anticipation and vulnerability.

- **At-Home Insemination:** Couples may choose to roleplay a more intimate setting, where they prepare for an insemination at home. This can include discussions about timing, selecting the right sperm donor, and the emotional implications of the process. The intimacy of this setting can enhance the connection between partners.

- **The Thrill of the Unknown:** Incorporating an element of surprise can heighten the excitement. For instance, one partner may not know when the insemination will occur, creating an atmosphere of suspense and desire.

The Thrill of Insemination Fantasies

Fantasizing about artificial insemination can evoke a range of emotions and desires. It can tap into themes of control, power dynamics, and vulnerability. For some, the idea of being inseminated can be a profound expression of trust and intimacy. The anticipation of waiting for the results can also create a sense of longing and excitement.

Exploring Different Methods and Tools

In the context of roleplay, various methods and tools can be utilized to enhance the experience of artificial insemination. Some of these may include:

- **Syringes and Catheters:** Utilizing medical tools can add authenticity to the roleplay. These items can be used to simulate the insemination process, allowing partners to engage in the act with a sense of realism.

- **Sperm Samples:** Using realistic sperm samples, such as artificial sperm or other fluids, can enhance the sensory experience. This can also include discussions about the donor's characteristics, further enriching the fantasy.

- **Fertility Monitors:** Incorporating fertility tracking devices can add an element of preparation and anticipation. This can involve roleplaying the monitoring of ovulation and discussing the optimal timing for insemination.

Medical Play and Fetishization

Artificial insemination naturally lends itself to medical play, which is a popular kink within the BDSM community. The clinical aspects of the procedure can be fetishized, and roleplay can explore themes of power exchange between the medical professional and the patient.

In these scenarios, the medical professional may exert control over the process, while the patient may experience a blend of vulnerability and excitement. This dynamic can create a rich tapestry of emotions and desires that enhances the overall experience.

Psychological Aspects of Artificial Insemination Roleplay

Engaging in artificial insemination roleplay can evoke various psychological responses, including feelings of empowerment, vulnerability, and intimacy. The act of insemination can symbolize a deep connection between partners, as it often involves discussions about future family planning and shared desires.

However, it is crucial to approach these scenarios with care, as they may trigger emotional responses related to fertility issues or past experiences. Open communication and consent are essential to navigate these complexities effectively.

Incorporating Themes of Dominance and Submission

Artificial insemination roleplay can also explore themes of dominance and submission. The dominant partner may take control of the insemination process, while the submissive partner may surrender to the experience. This dynamic can heighten the eroticism of the scenario, as power exchange becomes a central theme.

In these situations, clear boundaries and consent are paramount to ensure that both partners feel safe and respected. Establishing safewords and check-ins can help navigate the emotional landscape of this roleplay effectively.

Exploring the Emotions of Fertility Treatment

Incorporating artificial insemination into erotic roleplay can also provide an opportunity to explore the emotional aspects of fertility treatments. Couples may find themselves navigating feelings of hope, anxiety, and longing as they engage in this process.

Roleplay can serve as a safe space to express these emotions and fantasies, allowing partners to connect on a deeper level. It can also provide an avenue for discussing real-life experiences and feelings surrounding fertility, creating a sense of intimacy and understanding.

Conclusion

Artificial insemination offers a unique and multifaceted avenue for exploration within breeding fantasies and erotic roleplay. By understanding the techniques, psychological implications, and emotional dynamics involved, partners can engage in this theme with creativity and care. As with any roleplay scenario, prioritizing consent, communication, and emotional well-being is essential to ensure a fulfilling and enriching experience for both partners.

Understanding the process of artificial insemination

Artificial insemination (AI) is a medical procedure that involves the deliberate introduction of sperm into a female's reproductive system for the purpose of achieving pregnancy without sexual intercourse. This method is widely used in various contexts, including fertility treatments for couples facing challenges in conception, single women wishing to conceive, and same-sex couples seeking to start a family. Understanding the process of artificial insemination requires an exploration of its methodology, types, and the psychological implications associated with it.

Types of Artificial Insemination

There are primarily two types of artificial insemination:

- **Intrauterine Insemination (IUI):** This method involves placing sperm directly into the uterus using a thin catheter. IUI is often preferred for its higher success rates compared to other methods, as it allows sperm to bypass the cervix and reach the uterus more directly.

- **Intracervical Insemination (ICI):** In this method, sperm is deposited directly into the cervix. ICI is less invasive than IUI and can be performed at home with the right tools, making it a popular choice for individuals who prefer privacy and comfort.

The Process of Artificial Insemination

The process of artificial insemination can be broken down into several key steps:

1. **Sperm Collection:** Sperm can be collected from a partner or a sperm donor. In the case of donor sperm, it is usually obtained from a sperm bank where it is screened for health and genetic factors.

2. **Sperm Preparation:** The collected sperm is processed to separate motile sperm from seminal fluid and other non-motile sperm. This is typically done through a technique called sperm washing, which enhances the chances of successful fertilization.

3. **Timing of Insemination:** To maximize the chances of conception, insemination is timed to coincide with the female's ovulation. This may involve tracking ovulation through various methods, such as ovulation predictor kits or monitoring basal body temperature.

4. **Insemination Procedure:** Depending on the chosen method (IUI or ICI), the sperm is introduced into the reproductive tract. For IUI, a healthcare professional will perform the procedure in a clinical setting, while ICI can be performed at home.

5. **Post-Insemination Monitoring**: After insemination, the individual may be advised to rest for a short period. A pregnancy test is usually conducted a couple of weeks later to determine if the procedure was successful.

Psychological Aspects and Considerations

The psychological implications of artificial insemination can be profound. Individuals undergoing AI may experience a range of emotions, including hope, anxiety, and fear of failure. The anticipation of pregnancy can be both exhilarating and stressful, as the success of the procedure is often uncertain.

Moreover, the choice of a sperm donor can also bring about complex feelings. Considerations regarding the donor's characteristics, health history, and the potential for future contact can weigh heavily on the minds of those involved. It is crucial for individuals and couples to engage in open discussions about their feelings and expectations surrounding the process.

Ethical and Social Considerations

Artificial insemination raises several ethical and social questions. The selection of sperm donors, for instance, can lead to discussions about genetic diversity and the implications of donor anonymity. Furthermore, the rights of donors, recipients, and any resulting offspring can complicate relationships and societal norms.

In some cultures, AI may face stigma, particularly in contexts where traditional notions of family and reproduction prevail. Addressing societal judgments and fostering supportive environments for those exploring AI is essential for promoting acceptance and understanding.

Conclusion

Understanding the process of artificial insemination encompasses not only the technical aspects of the procedure but also the emotional, ethical, and social dimensions that accompany it. As more individuals and couples turn to AI as a means of achieving parenthood, it is vital to approach the topic with sensitivity and awareness of the diverse experiences involved.

$$\text{Success Rate} = \frac{\text{Number of Successful Pregnancies}}{\text{Total Inseminations}} \times 100\% \qquad (4)$$

The success rates of artificial insemination can vary based on numerous factors including the age of the individual, underlying fertility issues, and the method used. Generally, IUI has a success rate of approximately 10-20% per cycle, while ICI may have lower rates due to the less direct introduction of sperm.

In conclusion, artificial insemination is a multifaceted process that requires careful consideration of various factors to ensure a positive experience for all parties involved. As societal perspectives on family and reproduction continue to evolve, so too will the conversations surrounding artificial insemination and its role in modern parenthood.

Roleplaying insemination techniques

Roleplaying insemination techniques can be an exhilarating and intimate aspect of breeding fantasy. This section explores various methods and scenarios that can enhance the experience while ensuring safety and consent are prioritized.

Understanding Insemination Techniques

Insemination refers to the introduction of sperm into the female reproductive system for the purpose of achieving pregnancy. In roleplay, this can take on various forms, each with its unique appeal and emotional resonance.

Natural Insemination Natural insemination is the most straightforward method, involving penetrative intercourse where the goal is to conceive. Roleplaying this scenario can involve exploring the anticipation and excitement that comes with the act of trying to conceive. Partners may engage in discussions about ovulation cycles, fertility windows, and the intimate connection that comes from the act itself.

Artificial Insemination Artificial insemination, on the other hand, involves the use of medical techniques to introduce sperm into the reproductive tract. This can include:

- **Intracervical Insemination (ICI):** Involves placing sperm directly into the cervix.

- **Intrauterine Insemination (IUI):** Involves placing sperm directly into the uterus using a catheter.

- **Intravaginal Insemination (IVI):** Involves placing sperm in the vagina, relying on the body's natural processes for conception.

Each method can be roleplayed with varying degrees of realism, from using props to simulate medical equipment to employing narrative techniques that enhance the emotional depth of the experience.

Creating the Scene

When roleplaying insemination techniques, creating an immersive environment is key. Here are some elements to consider:

Setting The setting can significantly influence the experience. A clinical environment, such as a doctor's office or a home setting designed to mimic a medical procedure, can create a sense of authenticity. Alternatively, a more intimate setting can enhance the emotional connection between partners.

Props and Tools Using props can enhance the realism of the roleplay. For example:

- **Syringes or Catheters:** These can be used to simulate the artificial insemination process.

- **Lubricants:** Various lubricants can be used to enhance comfort and realism during the act.

- **Fertility Monitors or Ovulation Kits:** These props can add to the narrative by highlighting the planning involved in conception.

Communication and Consent

Before engaging in roleplay involving insemination techniques, it is crucial to have open and honest communication. Partners should discuss:

- **Boundaries:** Clearly define what is acceptable and what is off-limits.

- **Safewords:** Establish safewords to ensure that both partners can pause or stop the roleplay if it becomes uncomfortable.

- **Emotional Triggers:** Discuss any potential emotional triggers related to the themes of fertility, conception, or medical procedures.

Emotional Dynamics

Roleplaying insemination techniques can evoke a range of emotions, from excitement to anxiety. It is essential to address these feelings openly. Consider the following:

Anticipation and Anxiety The anticipation of conception can be thrilling, but it can also bring anxiety, especially if there are real-life concerns about fertility or pregnancy. Partners should support each other emotionally, discussing their feelings before and after the roleplay.

Aftercare Aftercare is an essential component of any roleplay scenario, particularly those that involve intense emotions. This can include physical comfort, such as cuddling or soothing words, as well as discussing the experience to ensure both partners feel satisfied and secure.

Examples of Roleplay Scenarios

Here are some examples of roleplaying scenarios involving insemination techniques:

Scenario 1: The Fertility Clinic In this scenario, one partner plays the role of a fertility specialist, while the other is the patient. The "doctor" prepares the "patient" for an insemination procedure, discussing the process and what to expect. This can include using props like medical instruments and discussing the emotional aspects of seeking fertility treatment.

Scenario 2: The Intimate Home Insemination In this scenario, partners create a private and intimate setting at home. They engage in discussions about their desire to conceive, followed by an artificial insemination process using props. This scenario can emphasize the emotional connection and intimacy involved in the act of trying to conceive.

Scenario 3: The Animalistic Breeding Fantasy In this scenario, partners can explore the primal aspects of breeding. One partner may take on a more dominant role, while the other submits to the act of insemination. This can include using animalistic language, sounds, and behaviors to enhance the fantasy.

Conclusion

Roleplaying insemination techniques offers a unique opportunity to explore the themes of fertility, intimacy, and desire within a safe and consensual framework. By understanding the various methods, creating immersive scenes, and maintaining open communication, partners can engage in fulfilling and exciting roleplay that deepens their connection and enhances their sexual experiences.

The thrill of insemination fantasies

Insemination fantasies encompass a wide range of erotic scenarios that revolve around the act of conceiving a child, often highlighting the excitement and allure of the process. This section delves into the psychological and emotional components that contribute to the thrill of these fantasies, as well as the various ways they can be explored in a consensual and safe manner.

Understanding Insemination Fantasies

At the core of insemination fantasies is the interplay of desire, power, and the biological imperative of reproduction. These fantasies often evoke feelings of intimacy and vulnerability, as they tap into deep-seated desires for connection and the creation of life. The thrill can be attributed to several factors:

- **Biological Urges:** The instinctual drive to reproduce is a powerful motivator that can manifest in sexual fantasies. This biological imperative can create a sense of urgency and excitement around the act of insemination.

- **Power Dynamics:** Insemination fantasies often involve elements of power exchange, where one partner assumes a dominant role while the other is submissive. This dynamic can heighten arousal and create a thrilling atmosphere of control and surrender.

- **Risk and Taboo:** Engaging in fantasies about insemination can evoke feelings of risk and taboo, particularly in societies where discussions of reproduction and sexuality are often shrouded in secrecy. This element of danger can amplify the excitement surrounding the fantasy.

- **Emotional Connection:** The act of insemination is inherently intimate, often requiring a deep emotional bond between partners. This connection can enhance the thrill, as partners explore their fantasies within a safe and trusting environment.

Exploring Insemination Fantasies

When exploring insemination fantasies, it is essential to approach them with care and consideration. Here are some methods to engage in these fantasies while maintaining a focus on consent and emotional well-being:

- **Roleplay Scenarios:** Couples can create detailed roleplay scenarios that incorporate insemination themes. For instance, one partner may take on the role of a fertility doctor, while the other plays the patient. This can introduce elements of medical play, heightening the sense of realism and excitement.

- **Use of Props:** Incorporating props such as syringes, vials, or even pregnancy-related items can enhance the sensory experience of the fantasy. These props can serve as tangible reminders of the fantasy, making it feel more immersive.

- **Storytelling:** Engaging in erotic storytelling can help partners articulate their desires and fantasies. By crafting narratives that revolve around insemination, individuals can explore their fantasies in a creative and intimate way.

- **Fantasy Journals:** Keeping a journal dedicated to insemination fantasies can provide a safe space for individuals to reflect on their desires, fears, and experiences. This practice can foster self-discovery and enhance communication between partners.

Addressing Challenges

While the thrill of insemination fantasies can be exhilarating, it is crucial to address potential challenges that may arise:

- **Emotional Triggers:** Insemination fantasies may evoke strong emotions, particularly for individuals who have experienced fertility struggles or pregnancy loss. It is vital to engage in open discussions about these feelings and establish boundaries to ensure emotional safety.

- **Consent and Communication:** Clear communication is essential when exploring insemination fantasies. Partners should discuss their boundaries, desires, and any potential triggers before engaging in roleplay or fantasy exploration.

- **Societal Stigma:** The taboo nature of insemination fantasies may lead to feelings of shame or guilt. It is important for individuals to recognize that their fantasies are valid and to seek supportive communities where they can share their experiences without judgment.

Conclusion

Insemination fantasies can be a thrilling and deeply intimate exploration of desire, power, and connection. By approaching these fantasies with care, consent, and open communication, individuals can create enriching experiences that enhance their sexual relationships. Whether through roleplay, storytelling, or the use of props, the thrill of insemination fantasies can be a fulfilling aspect of erotic life, inviting partners to explore the depths of their desires while fostering trust and intimacy.

$$\text{Thrill} = \text{Biological Urges} + \text{Power Dynamics} + \text{Risk} + \text{Emotional Connection} \quad (5)$$

Exploring different methods and tools

In the realm of breeding fantasies and erotic pregnancy play, the exploration of various methods and tools can significantly enhance the experience, making it more immersive and fulfilling. This section delves into the different approaches to roleplaying artificial insemination and conception, as well as the tools that can be utilized to create a more vivid and engaging fantasy.

Understanding Artificial Insemination Techniques

Artificial insemination (AI) is a medical procedure that involves the introduction of sperm into a woman's reproductive system by means other than sexual intercourse. In the context of erotic roleplay, this technique can be adapted to fit a variety of scenarios that cater to the fantasy of conception without the traditional act of intercourse.

Methods of Artificial Insemination There are several methods of artificial insemination that can be explored in roleplay scenarios:

- **Intracervical Insemination (ICI):** This method involves placing sperm directly into the cervix, allowing it to travel into the uterus. In roleplay, this can be simulated with the use of syringes or other medical tools to create a sense of realism.

- **Intrauterine Insemination (IUI):** In this method, sperm is placed directly into the uterus using a catheter. Roleplaying this scenario can involve the use of props that mimic medical instruments, thus enhancing the authenticity of the experience.

- **Intratubal Insemination (ITI):** This less common method involves placing sperm directly into the fallopian tubes. While it is less frequently used in roleplay, it can add an element of complexity to the scenario.

Tools and Props for Roleplay

Incorporating tools and props into breeding fantasies can elevate the experience, making it feel more tangible and exciting. Here are some tools that can be utilized in roleplay:

Medical Instruments Using medical instruments can enhance the realism of artificial insemination roleplay. Items such as:

- **Syringes:** These can be used to simulate the act of insemination, whether through ICI or IUI. They can be filled with various substances to heighten the fantasy.

- **Catheters:** For those roleplaying IUI, a catheter can be used to mimic the medical procedure, adding an element of authenticity.

- **Speculums:** Although primarily used in gynecological exams, incorporating a speculum can enhance the medical aspect of the fantasy, providing a sense of vulnerability and submission.

Fertility Tools In addition to medical instruments, various fertility tools can be used to create a more immersive experience:

- **Ovulation Predictor Kits:** These kits can be integrated into the roleplay to simulate the process of tracking ovulation and fertility. Characters can engage in discussions about timing and readiness, enhancing the anticipation.

- **Fertility Charts:** Creating a fertility chart can add a layer of planning and strategy to the roleplay, allowing participants to visualize the timing of insemination.

- **Fertility Supplements:** Incorporating discussions about fertility supplements or herbs can add depth to the roleplay, allowing for exploration of natural conception methods.

Psychological Aspects of Artificial Insemination Roleplay

The psychological aspect of engaging in artificial insemination roleplay is crucial to understanding its appeal. Participants may find themselves drawn to the themes of control, vulnerability, and intimacy that this type of roleplay can evoke.

Emotional Connection Artificial insemination roleplay can foster a deep emotional connection between partners. The act of insemination, whether simulated or real, can create a sense of shared purpose and intimacy. Participants may feel a heightened sense of closeness as they engage in discussions about their desires, boundaries, and fantasies.

Power Dynamics Exploring power dynamics is a significant aspect of breeding fantasies. In the context of artificial insemination roleplay, one partner may take on a more dominant role, while the other assumes a submissive position. This dynamic can enhance the thrill of the experience, as the dominant partner guides the submissive through the process, reinforcing feelings of trust and safety.

Fantasy vs. Reality It is essential to maintain a balance between fantasy and reality during roleplay. While the tools and methods used can enhance the experience, participants should be aware of their limits and the boundaries established prior to engaging in the fantasy. Open communication about feelings and experiences is crucial to ensure that both partners feel safe and fulfilled.

Incorporating Themes of Dominance and Submission

The themes of dominance and submission can be seamlessly woven into artificial insemination roleplay. This can be achieved through:

- **Role Assignment:** Assigning roles based on dominance and submission can add an exciting layer to the fantasy. The dominant partner may take charge of the insemination process, while the submissive partner may surrender control, heightening the emotional stakes.

- **Scripts and Scenarios:** Creating scripts that incorporate elements of power exchange can enhance the experience. For example, the dominant partner may dictate the terms of the insemination, while the submissive partner follows their lead.

- **Physical Restraints:** Incorporating physical restraints, such as cuffs or ropes, can further emphasize the power dynamics at play. This can create a heightened sense of vulnerability for the submissive partner, enhancing the erotic nature of the fantasy.

Conclusion

Exploring different methods and tools in breeding fantasies, particularly in the context of artificial insemination, can significantly enrich the experience for participants. By understanding the various techniques available, utilizing props and instruments, and incorporating psychological and power dynamics, partners can create a deeply immersive and fulfilling roleplay scenario. The key lies in communication, consent, and a shared understanding of boundaries, ensuring that the fantasy remains a safe and enjoyable exploration of desire.

Medical Play and Fetishization

Medical play is a form of roleplay that incorporates elements of medical scenarios into erotic fantasies. It often involves the use of medical instruments, uniforms, and procedures, creating a unique blend of arousal and vulnerability. This section explores the intersection of medical play and fetishization, examining the psychological underpinnings, potential issues, and practical examples.

Theoretical Background

The allure of medical play can be traced back to several psychological theories. One prominent theory is the **Conditioning Theory**, which suggests that individuals may develop a sexual response to medical environments due to early experiences or associations. For instance, a person who experienced a pleasurable or exciting event in a medical setting may later find themselves aroused by similar scenarios.

Additionally, **Power Dynamics** play a crucial role in medical fetishization. The roles of doctor and patient inherently involve a power imbalance, which can be both thrilling and comforting for participants. This dynamic allows individuals to explore themes of dominance and submission, heightening the erotic experience.

Common Themes in Medical Play

+ **Examinations:** Roleplaying medical examinations can evoke feelings of vulnerability and trust. The act of being examined can serve as a powerful metaphor for intimacy.

+ **Procedures:** Fantasies involving medical procedures—such as injections or surgeries—can heighten excitement through the anticipation of the unknown.

+ **Uniforms and Instruments:** The visual and tactile elements of medical uniforms (e.g., lab coats, scrubs) and instruments (e.g., stethoscopes, syringes) can enhance the fetishization of the experience.

Potential Problems and Ethical Considerations

While medical play can be a thrilling exploration of fantasy, it is essential to navigate potential problems and ethical concerns:

+ **Consent and Safety:** Clear communication and consent are paramount. Participants should establish boundaries and ensure that all activities are safe and consensual.

+ **Real-life Trauma:** For some individuals, medical scenarios may trigger past trauma related to healthcare experiences. It is crucial to be aware of and sensitive to these triggers.

+ **Legal and Social Implications:** Engaging in medical play may raise legal questions, especially if it involves the use of real medical instruments or settings. Participants must be mindful of local laws and societal perceptions.

Examples of Medical Play Scenarios

1. **The Check-Up:**

    + One partner takes on the role of a doctor, while the other plays the patient. The doctor conducts a thorough examination, incorporating playful dialogue and physical examination techniques.

2. **The Injection:**

- This scenario involves the administering of an injection, using a prop syringe. The anticipation of the "injection" can create an exhilarating sense of vulnerability.

3. **The Surgery:**

- Participants can roleplay a surgical procedure, with one partner acting as the surgeon and the other as the patient. This scenario can involve props like surgical masks and instruments to enhance realism.

Conclusion

Medical play and fetishization offer a unique avenue for exploring power dynamics, vulnerability, and intimacy within erotic contexts. By understanding the psychological underpinnings and addressing potential concerns, individuals can safely and consensually engage in these fantasies, enriching their sexual experiences and deepening their connections with partners.

Psychological aspects of artificial insemination roleplay

Artificial insemination roleplay is a nuanced and multifaceted area of erotic fantasy that intertwines with various psychological themes. Understanding these psychological aspects is crucial for participants to navigate their fantasies safely and meaningfully. This section delves into the psychological implications of engaging in artificial insemination roleplay, including identity exploration, power dynamics, emotional responses, and the intersection of fantasy with reality.

Identity Exploration

One of the most profound psychological aspects of artificial insemination roleplay is the exploration of identity. Participants may find themselves grappling with their desires, roles, and the implications of parenthood. This exploration can manifest in several ways:

- **Parental Identity:** Engaging in this roleplay may allow individuals to explore their feelings about becoming parents, whether they are interested in parenting or are ambivalent. The act of roleplaying insemination can evoke a sense of nurturing or caretaking, which can be both exhilarating and daunting.

- **Gender Roles and Expectations:** This roleplay often brings to the surface societal expectations regarding gender and parenting. Participants may find themselves questioning traditional roles, allowing for the exploration of non-binary identities or alternative family structures.

- **Personal Fantasies:** Participants can explore their fantasies surrounding fertility, motherhood, and family dynamics, which may differ significantly from their real-life situations. This exploration can lead to a deeper understanding of personal desires and motivations.

Power Dynamics

Artificial insemination roleplay often involves complex power dynamics that can heighten the erotic experience. Understanding these dynamics is essential for ensuring a consensual and fulfilling experience:

- **Dominance and Submission:** Many participants find the interplay of dominance and submission within the context of artificial insemination particularly stimulating. The dominant partner may take on the role of the inseminator, while the submissive partner may embody the receptive role. This dynamic can create a heightened sense of vulnerability and trust, which can be incredibly erotic.

- **Control and Surrender:** The act of roleplaying artificial insemination often involves themes of control and surrender. The submissive partner may experience a release of control by allowing the dominant partner to take the lead in the insemination process. This surrender can be liberating and deeply fulfilling, tapping into primal instincts and desires.

- **Negotiation of Power:** The negotiation of power dynamics is critical in ensuring that both partners feel safe and respected. Open communication about desires, boundaries, and limits is essential to navigate these dynamics effectively.

Emotional Responses

Engaging in artificial insemination roleplay can evoke a wide range of emotional responses, which can enhance or complicate the experience:

- **Excitement and Anticipation:** The thrill of engaging in a fantasy that involves conception can generate excitement and anticipation. The buildup to the act can heighten arousal and create a sense of urgency that enhances the overall experience.

+ **Fear and Anxiety:** For some, the themes of artificial insemination may trigger fears or anxieties related to pregnancy, parenthood, or fertility issues. It is essential to address these feelings openly and honestly, allowing partners to support each other through any emotional turbulence.

+ **Joy and Fulfillment:** Successfully navigating the roleplay can lead to feelings of joy and fulfillment. Participants may experience a sense of accomplishment in exploring their fantasies and desires, leading to deeper intimacy and connection with their partner.

Fantasy vs. Reality

The line between fantasy and reality can become blurred in artificial insemination roleplay, leading to potential psychological challenges:

+ **Escapism:** Roleplay can serve as a form of escapism, allowing participants to temporarily step away from their everyday lives and immerse themselves in their fantasies. However, it is crucial to maintain a balance between fantasy and reality to avoid disillusionment or dissatisfaction with real-life relationships.

+ **Fear of Consequences:** The potential consequences of artificial insemination, such as pregnancy or emotional attachment, can create anxiety for participants. Open communication about these fears is vital to ensure that both partners feel secure in their roles.

+ **Integration of Experiences:** Participants should consider how their experiences within the roleplay may impact their real-life relationships and desires. Reflecting on these experiences can lead to personal growth and a deeper understanding of one's identity and desires.

Conclusion

The psychological aspects of artificial insemination roleplay are intricate and deeply personal. By understanding the themes of identity exploration, power dynamics, emotional responses, and the interplay between fantasy and reality, participants can engage in this roleplay more meaningfully and safely. Prioritizing open communication, consent, and emotional support will ensure that the experience is fulfilling and enriching, allowing individuals to explore their desires in a safe and consensual environment.

Incorporating themes of dominance and submission

In the realm of breeding fantasy, the interplay of dominance and submission (D/s) adds a complex layer of psychological and emotional engagement. This dynamic can enhance the erotic experience, allowing participants to explore power exchange in a safe and consensual environment. Understanding the theoretical underpinnings of D/s relationships is crucial for integrating these themes into breeding roleplay scenarios.

Theoretical Framework

Dominance and submission can be analyzed through various psychological lenses, including social dominance theory, attachment theory, and the BDSM framework. Social dominance theory posits that social hierarchies are formed based on power dynamics, which can manifest in intimate relationships. In the context of breeding fantasy, the dominant partner often embodies the archetype of the provider or protector, while the submissive partner may adopt a more vulnerable, receptive role.

Attachment theory further illustrates how individuals relate to one another based on their early experiences with caregivers. Those with secure attachments may navigate D/s dynamics with ease, while those with anxious or avoidant attachments may experience challenges. Understanding these dynamics is essential for establishing trust and safety in breeding roleplay.

The BDSM framework offers a structured approach to exploring D/s relationships, emphasizing the importance of consent, negotiation, and communication. Participants are encouraged to discuss their desires, limits, and safe words before engaging in roleplay, ensuring that both parties feel empowered and respected.

Common Problems and Solutions

While the incorporation of D/s themes can be thrilling, it is not without potential pitfalls. Common challenges include miscommunication, power imbalances, and emotional triggers. To mitigate these issues, partners should prioritize ongoing communication and establish clear boundaries.

- **Miscommunication:** Participants may have different interpretations of dominance and submission. To address this, engage in open discussions about what D/s means to each partner, including specific actions, language, and expectations.

- **Power Imbalances:** It is vital to ensure that the dominant partner does not exploit their power. Regular check-ins during roleplay can help maintain a balance of power and ensure that the submissive partner feels safe and respected.

- **Emotional Triggers:** Breeding fantasies can evoke strong emotions, particularly if they touch on past experiences. Partners should be aware of each other's emotional triggers and have strategies in place for managing them, such as pausing the scene or incorporating aftercare.

Practical Examples

Incorporating D/s themes into breeding fantasies can take various forms, each tailored to the preferences and comfort levels of the participants. Here are some practical examples:

1. **Role Reversal:** In a roleplay scenario, the dominant partner may take on the role of a doctor or fertility specialist, guiding the submissive partner through a simulated insemination process. This dynamic allows the submissive to explore vulnerability while the dominant exerts control over the situation.

2. **Ritualistic Breeding Contracts:** Couples can create a symbolic breeding contract that outlines the terms of their roleplay. This contract can include specific behaviors, safewords, and aftercare protocols, reinforcing the D/s dynamic while emphasizing consent and mutual agreement.

3. **Training Scenarios:** The dominant partner may engage in "training" the submissive to prepare for pregnancy, incorporating tasks that emphasize obedience and submission. This could involve the submissive following specific routines or rituals that heighten their anticipation of becoming pregnant.

Conclusion

Incorporating themes of dominance and submission into breeding fantasy can enrich the erotic experience, allowing participants to explore power dynamics in a consensual and safe manner. By understanding the theoretical frameworks, addressing potential challenges, and implementing practical examples, couples can create fulfilling and empowering breeding roleplay scenarios. As always, the cornerstone of this exploration lies in open communication, trust, and mutual respect, ensuring that both partners feel valued and heard throughout their journey.

Exploring the emotions of fertility treatment

Fertility treatment can evoke a complex array of emotions, ranging from hope and excitement to anxiety, frustration, and grief. Understanding these emotions is crucial for individuals and couples navigating the often challenging journey of conception. This section delves into the psychological landscape of fertility treatment, exploring common emotional responses, the impact of these emotions on relationships, and strategies for managing emotional well-being throughout the process.

The Emotional Rollercoaster

Fertility treatment typically involves various medical interventions, such as in vitro fertilization (IVF), intrauterine insemination (IUI), or hormone therapy. Each stage of treatment can trigger different emotional responses, including:

- **Hope and Anticipation:** Initially, individuals may feel a sense of hope as they embark on the treatment journey. The prospect of becoming parents can be exhilarating, fostering a sense of excitement about the future.

- **Anxiety and Stress:** As treatment progresses, anxiety often escalates. Concerns about the effectiveness of the treatment, potential side effects, and the financial burden can create significant stress. The uncertainty of outcomes can lead to feelings of helplessness.

- **Frustration and Disappointment:** If treatment cycles do not yield the desired results, frustration can set in. Each failed attempt may feel like a setback, leading to feelings of inadequacy or self-blame.

- **Grief and Loss:** Many individuals experience grief related to their fertility struggles. This grief may stem from the loss of the idealized vision of parenthood or from unsuccessful treatment attempts. It is essential to acknowledge and process these feelings of loss.

- **Isolation and Loneliness:** The emotional burden of fertility treatment can lead to feelings of isolation. Individuals may feel that others do not understand their struggles, which can exacerbate feelings of loneliness.

Impact on Relationships

The emotional toll of fertility treatment can significantly impact relationships. Partners may react differently to the stress of treatment, leading to misunderstandings and conflicts. Common relationship challenges include:

- **Communication Breakdowns:** Stress and anxiety can hinder open communication. Partners may struggle to express their feelings, leading to a disconnect in emotional intimacy.

- **Role Reversal:** Traditional gender roles may shift during treatment, with one partner taking on a more nurturing role while the other feels pressured to provide emotional support. This shift can create tension and resentment.

- **Intimacy Issues:** The clinical nature of fertility treatments can diminish sexual intimacy. Couples may find it challenging to engage in spontaneous sexual activity, leading to feelings of pressure and performance anxiety.

- **Support and Understanding:** On the other hand, navigating fertility treatment together can strengthen a relationship. Couples who communicate openly and support each other through the process often report increased intimacy and bonding.

Coping Strategies

To navigate the emotional complexities of fertility treatment, individuals and couples can adopt various coping strategies:

- **Open Communication:** Establishing a safe space for open dialogue is crucial. Partners should share their feelings, fears, and hopes, fostering emotional intimacy and understanding.

- **Seek Professional Support:** Engaging with mental health professionals, such as therapists specializing in fertility issues, can provide valuable support. Therapy can help individuals process their emotions and develop healthy coping mechanisms.

- **Join Support Groups:** Connecting with others who are experiencing similar challenges can alleviate feelings of isolation. Support groups provide a space for sharing experiences, advice, and emotional support.

- **Practice Self-Care:** Prioritizing self-care is essential for emotional well-being. Activities such as exercise, meditation, and hobbies can help reduce stress and promote emotional balance.

- **Set Realistic Expectations:** Understanding that fertility treatment can be unpredictable helps manage expectations. Couples should approach each treatment cycle with a realistic mindset, recognizing that outcomes may vary.

Conclusion

Exploring the emotions surrounding fertility treatment is vital for individuals and couples engaged in this journey. By recognizing and addressing the emotional challenges, partners can cultivate a supportive environment that fosters intimacy and resilience. While the path to parenthood may be fraught with difficulties, understanding the emotional landscape can empower individuals to navigate their experiences with compassion and grace. The journey may be long and arduous, but with the right support and coping strategies, hope can prevail, illuminating the path toward parenthood.

Breeding fetish

Breeding fetish, a specific subset of erotic fantasy, revolves around the desire for reproduction and the act of insemination, often tied to themes of fertility, dominance, and submission. This phenomenon is characterized by a complex interplay of biological impulses, psychological needs, and societal taboos. Understanding breeding fetish requires delving into the motivations behind it, the dynamics of power involved, and the ways in which individuals navigate their fantasies within the context of real-life relationships.

Defining Breeding Fetish

At its core, breeding fetish is defined by a heightened interest in the act of conception, the physical and emotional aspects of pregnancy, and the implications of creating life. For many, this fetish is not merely about the act itself but encompasses a broader narrative that includes themes of fertility, nurturing, and the primal instincts associated with reproduction.

The Psychological Appeal

The psychological appeal of breeding fetish can be traced to several factors:

- **Biological Imperatives:** The drive to reproduce is a fundamental aspect of human nature. Breeding fetish taps into this primal urge, allowing individuals to explore their biological instincts in a safe and consensual manner.

- **Power Dynamics:** Breeding scenarios often involve clear power exchanges, where one partner assumes a dominant role while the other is submissive. This dynamic can heighten arousal and create a sense of safety and surrender for both parties.

- **Nurturing and Care:** The themes of nurturing and care associated with pregnancy can evoke feelings of warmth and intimacy, making breeding fetish a deeply emotional experience.

Common Scenarios in Breeding Fetish

Breeding fetish can manifest in various roleplay scenarios, each tailored to the desires and boundaries of the participants. Some common scenarios include:

- **Natural Conception:** Roleplaying the act of natural conception can involve explicit discussions about fertility cycles, ovulation, and the excitement of trying to conceive. This scenario often emphasizes the intimacy and connection between partners.

- **Medical Play:** Incorporating elements of medical play, such as fertility treatments or insemination procedures, can add a layer of realism and excitement. This may involve the use of props or tools that simulate medical environments.

- **Animalistic Dynamics:** Some individuals explore their breeding fetish through animalistic themes, embracing primal instincts and behaviors. This could involve roleplaying as animals or using language that reflects a more instinctual approach to reproduction.

- **Fantasy and Storytelling:** Creating elaborate narratives around breeding scenarios can enhance the experience. This may include crafting backstories, character development, and setting the scene for the fantasy to unfold.

The Role of Consent and Communication

As with any fetish or roleplay scenario, consent and communication are paramount in breeding fetish. Participants should engage in open discussions about their desires, boundaries, and any potential triggers before embarking on their exploration.

$$C = \frac{D + B + T}{R} \quad (6)$$

Where:

- C = Clarity of consent
- D = Desire for the scenario
- B = Boundaries established
- T = Trust between partners
- R = Realistic expectations

This equation illustrates that clarity of consent is achieved when desire, boundaries, and trust are balanced against realistic expectations of the roleplay.

Addressing Potential Problems

While breeding fetish can be a fulfilling exploration, it is essential to address potential problems that may arise:

- **Emotional Triggers:** Participants should be aware of any emotional triggers that may surface during roleplay, particularly those related to personal experiences with pregnancy, loss, or fertility issues.
- **Societal Stigma:** Breeding fetish may carry societal stigma, leading individuals to feel shame or embarrassment. Engaging in supportive communities or seeking therapy can help navigate these feelings.
- **Real-Life Implications:** It is crucial to differentiate between fantasy and reality. Participants should regularly check in with each other to ensure that their exploration remains consensual and enjoyable.

Exploring Breeding Communities

Many individuals find solace and understanding within breeding communities, both online and offline. These communities provide a space for sharing experiences, discussing fantasies, and connecting with like-minded individuals. Engaging with such communities can foster a sense of belonging and validation, allowing participants to explore their breeding fetish in a supportive environment.

Conclusion

Breeding fetish is a multifaceted exploration of desire, power dynamics, and the primal instincts associated with reproduction. By understanding the psychological appeal, engaging in open communication, and navigating potential challenges, individuals can create fulfilling and consensual breeding fantasies that enhance their intimate lives. As society continues to evolve in its understanding of sexuality and fetishism, breeding fetish can serve as a powerful avenue for self-discovery and connection between partners.

Anatomy and physiology of breeding

Breeding, in the context of erotic pregnancy play, encompasses a complex interplay of anatomical structures and physiological processes that facilitate reproduction. Understanding these elements is crucial for those engaging in breeding fantasies, as it deepens the experience and enhances the connection between partners.

The Female Reproductive System

The female reproductive system is designed for the processes of ovulation, fertilization, and gestation. Key components include:

- **Ovaries:** These are the primary reproductive organs that produce ova (eggs) and hormones such as estrogen and progesterone. Each month, during the menstrual cycle, an ovary releases an egg in a process known as ovulation.

- **Fallopian Tubes:** These tubes transport the egg from the ovaries to the uterus. Fertilization typically occurs within the fallopian tubes when sperm meets the egg.

- **Uterus:** A muscular organ that provides a nurturing environment for a fertilized egg to implant and develop into a fetus. The lining of the uterus, known as the endometrium, thickens in preparation for potential implantation.

- **Cervix:** The lower part of the uterus that opens into the vagina. It plays a crucial role during pregnancy by producing mucus that can either facilitate or inhibit sperm passage depending on the menstrual cycle phase.
- **Vagina:** The canal that connects the external genitalia to the uterus. It serves as the passageway for sperm to enter the uterus and for childbirth.

The Male Reproductive System

The male reproductive system is equally important in the breeding process, with its main components being:

- **Testes:** These organs produce sperm and testosterone. Sperm production occurs in the seminiferous tubules within the testes.
- **Epididymis:** A coiled structure where sperm mature and are stored.
- **Vas Deferens:** A duct that transports sperm from the epididymis to the ejaculatory duct during ejaculation.
- **Seminal Vesicles and Prostate Gland:** These glands produce seminal fluid, which nourishes and helps transport sperm during ejaculation.
- **Penis:** The external organ that delivers sperm into the female reproductive tract. Erection occurs through the engorgement of erectile tissue with blood, facilitating penetration.

The Process of Fertilization

Fertilization occurs when a sperm cell successfully penetrates an egg. This process can be broken down into several stages:

1. **Sperm Activation:** Upon ejaculation, sperm become motile and begin their journey through the female reproductive tract.
2. **Capacitation:** This is a biochemical process that sperm undergo to gain the ability to fertilize an egg, which occurs in the female reproductive system.
3. **Acrosome Reaction:** When a sperm reaches the egg, it releases enzymes from its acrosome, allowing it to penetrate the outer layers of the egg.

4. **Fusion:** Once a sperm penetrates the egg, the genetic materials combine, resulting in a zygote.

The successful fusion of sperm and egg marks the beginning of a new life, and this moment is often a focal point in breeding fantasies.

Hormonal Regulation in Breeding

Hormones play a pivotal role in regulating the reproductive cycle and facilitating breeding. Key hormones include:

- **Follicle-Stimulating Hormone (FSH):** Stimulates the growth of ovarian follicles in females and sperm production in males.

- **Luteinizing Hormone (LH):** Triggers ovulation and stimulates testosterone production in males.

- **Estrogen:** Regulates the menstrual cycle and prepares the uterus for potential pregnancy.

- **Progesterone:** Maintains the uterine lining for implantation and supports early pregnancy.

The interplay of these hormones creates a cyclical rhythm, influencing not only biological processes but also emotional and psychological states associated with breeding fantasies.

Anatomical Considerations in Breeding Roleplay

When engaging in breeding fantasies, individuals may explore various anatomical considerations to enhance the experience:

- **Positioning:** Certain sexual positions may be favored for their perceived effectiveness in facilitating conception, such as missionary or doggy style.

- **Sensory Experiences:** Incorporating elements that heighten awareness of anatomy, such as the warmth and texture of skin, can enhance arousal and connection.

- **Fertility Awareness:** Understanding the menstrual cycle, including ovulation timing, can add a layer of realism to roleplay scenarios.

Potential Problems and Considerations

While exploring breeding fantasies, individuals should be aware of potential problems that may arise:

- **Emotional Impact:** Engaging in breeding play may trigger strong emotions related to fertility, loss, or personal experiences. Open communication is essential to navigate these feelings.

- **Health Risks:** Participants should consider the implications of unprotected sex, including sexually transmitted infections (STIs) and unintended pregnancies. Safe practices should always be prioritized.

- **Consent and Boundaries:** Establishing clear boundaries and ensuring ongoing consent is paramount, especially given the sensitive nature of breeding fantasies.

Conclusion

Understanding the anatomy and physiology of breeding enriches the erotic experience of pregnancy play. By acknowledging the biological processes, hormonal influences, and emotional implications, participants can create a more profound connection within their fantasies. As with all aspects of erotic roleplay, safety, consent, and communication remain the cornerstones of a fulfilling experience.

$$\text{Fertility Rate} = \frac{\text{Number of Live Births}}{\text{Population of Women Aged 15-49}} \times 1000 \qquad (7)$$

This equation serves as a reminder of the biological realities underlying the fantasies, offering a bridge between the erotic and the empirical in the realm of breeding play.

Animalistic aspects of breeding fetish

The concept of breeding fetish often intersects with primal urges and animalistic instincts, tapping into deep-seated biological and psychological drives. This section explores the animalistic aspects of breeding fetish, delving into the underlying theories, potential problems, and illustrative examples that encapsulate this intriguing facet of erotic roleplay.

Theoretical Framework

Breeding fetishism can be understood through various theoretical lenses, including evolutionary psychology, psychoanalysis, and social constructivism. From an evolutionary perspective, the drive to reproduce is fundamentally linked to survival and the continuation of one's genetic lineage. As such, breeding fantasies may evoke a return to primal instincts that prioritize reproduction as a primary goal.

$$F = \frac{G \cdot m_1 \cdot m_2}{r^2} \qquad (8)$$

In this equation, F represents the gravitational force that binds individuals in a reproductive context, where G is the gravitational constant, m_1 and m_2 are the masses of the individuals involved, and r is the distance between them. This analogy illustrates how attraction can be seen as a force that draws individuals together, reminiscent of animal mating behaviors.

Psychoanalytic theory posits that breeding fetishes may stem from repressed desires and childhood experiences. Sigmund Freud's theories of sexuality suggest that our early relationships and experiences shape our adult desires. The animalistic aspect of breeding can evoke feelings of dominance, submission, and the raw, unfiltered nature of sexual attraction, reminiscent of animal mating rituals.

Animalistic Behaviors in Breeding Fantasy

Animalistic behaviors in breeding fetish often manifest through roleplay scenarios that mimic the mating rituals observed in the animal kingdom. For instance, participants may adopt specific roles that reflect predator-prey dynamics, where one partner embodies the dominant, assertive figure while the other assumes a more submissive, receptive role.

- **Predator-Prey Dynamics:** In this scenario, the dominant partner may use language and actions that reflect a hunting or stalking behavior, enhancing the thrill of the chase. The submissive partner may respond with a mix of fear and excitement, mirroring the instinctual responses seen in nature.

- **Pack Mentality:** Some individuals may explore breeding fantasies within a group context, emulating the social structures found in certain animal species. This can involve multiple partners and the dynamics of competition for mating rights, echoing the rituals of animals such as wolves or lions.

Problems and Considerations

While engaging in breeding fetish roleplay, it's crucial to be aware of potential problems that may arise from the animalistic aspects of these fantasies. Issues related to consent, boundaries, and emotional well-being must be addressed to ensure a safe and fulfilling experience.

- **Consent and Power Dynamics:** The primal nature of breeding fantasies can blur the lines of consent, particularly in scenarios that involve dominance and submission. Clear communication and the establishment of safewords are essential to navigate these dynamics safely.

- **Emotional Triggers:** Participants may encounter emotional triggers related to past experiences or societal norms surrounding reproduction. It is vital to engage in open discussions about these triggers and how they may impact the roleplay experience.

- **Social Stigma:** The animalistic aspects of breeding fetish may be met with societal judgment or misunderstanding. Participants should consider how to manage external perceptions and create a supportive environment for their exploration.

Examples of Animalistic Breeding Scenarios

To illustrate the animalistic aspects of breeding fetish, consider the following examples that highlight the interplay of instinctual behaviors and erotic roleplay:

1. **The Wild Encounter:** In this scenario, one partner takes on the role of a feral creature, embodying the raw, untamed aspects of nature. The other partner acts as a willing participant, drawn into the wildness of the encounter. The use of animalistic sounds, movements, and primal language enhances the immersive experience.

2. **The Alpha and the Omega:** This dynamic explores the hierarchy often seen in animal social structures. The dominant partner embodies the alpha figure, asserting control and guiding the submissive partner through the mating ritual. This scenario can involve elements of restraint and exploration of the submissive's limits, emphasizing trust and communication.

3. **Fertility Rituals:** Drawing inspiration from ancient practices, participants may engage in roleplay that mimics fertility rituals observed in various

cultures. These scenarios can include symbolic acts that celebrate reproduction, such as offerings, chants, or the use of props that represent fertility.

Conclusion

The animalistic aspects of breeding fetish provide a rich tapestry of exploration that intertwines primal instincts with erotic roleplay. By understanding the underlying theories, recognizing potential problems, and drawing upon illustrative examples, participants can navigate this complex terrain with awareness and care. Engaging in breeding fantasies that embrace these animalistic elements can lead to profound intimacy and connection, fostering a deeper understanding of oneself and one's desires within the context of consensual play.

Breeding as a power exchange

Breeding fantasies often intertwine with themes of power exchange, creating a unique and compelling dynamic that can deepen the intimacy and eroticism of the experience. This section explores the theoretical underpinnings of power dynamics in breeding scenarios, the potential challenges that may arise, and practical examples that illustrate these concepts.

Theoretical Framework

Power exchange in sexual relationships can be understood through the lens of Dominance and Submission (D/s) dynamics. In this context, one partner (the Dominant) exerts control over the other (the Submissive), which can manifest in various ways, including decision-making, physical restraint, or the establishment of specific roles within a fantasy.

Breeding fantasies amplify these dynamics by introducing elements of fertility, reproduction, and the potential for creating life. The Dominant may take on the role of the "sire," while the Submissive embodies the "breeder," creating a narrative where the act of conception is laden with power implications. This dynamic can be analyzed through the following theoretical frameworks:

- **Feminist Theory:** This perspective examines how power dynamics in breeding fantasies can reflect societal views on gender roles, reproduction, and sexuality. The Submissive's role as the potential mother can evoke traditional notions of femininity and domesticity, while the Dominant's role may reinforce patriarchal structures or challenge them through consensual roleplay.

- **Psychological Theory:** The psychological appeal of breeding fantasies often lies in the desire for connection, intimacy, and the exploration of vulnerability. The act of surrendering control to a partner can be deeply fulfilling, as it allows the Submissive to experience a sense of trust and safety within the confines of the fantasy.

- **Sociocultural Theory:** This framework examines how cultural narratives around reproduction and family influence individual desires and fantasies. Breeding as a power exchange can reflect personal and societal beliefs about parenthood, sexuality, and the roles of men and women in reproduction.

Challenges and Ethical Considerations

While breeding as a power exchange can be an exhilarating experience, it is essential to navigate potential challenges and ethical considerations. Some common issues include:

- **Consent and Communication:** Clear and ongoing communication is crucial when engaging in breeding fantasies. Partners must negotiate their desires, boundaries, and the extent of their roles within the power exchange. The use of safewords and regular check-ins can help ensure that both partners feel safe and respected throughout the experience.

- **Emotional Risks:** Engaging in breeding fantasies can evoke strong emotions, including feelings of vulnerability, anxiety, or even grief. It is essential for partners to discuss potential emotional triggers and establish aftercare practices to support one another after the roleplay.

- **Societal Judgment:** Breeding fantasies can be stigmatized, leading to feelings of shame or isolation. Partners must navigate societal perceptions and be prepared to face judgment from others. Establishing a supportive community or finding safe spaces for exploration can help mitigate these challenges.

Illustrative Examples

To further illustrate the concept of breeding as a power exchange, consider the following scenarios:

> **Example**
>
> **Scenario 1: The Fertility Ritual**
> In this roleplay, the Dominant creates a ritual around conception, establishing rules and guidelines for the Submissive to follow. The Dominant may instruct the Submissive to dress in specific clothing or engage in particular behaviors that enhance the fantasy of fertility. This power dynamic emphasizes the Dominant's control over the conception process while allowing the Submissive to embrace their role as the potential bearer of life.

> **Example**
>
> **Scenario 2: The Breeding Contract**
> Partners may choose to create a symbolic breeding contract that outlines the terms of their roleplay. This contract can include specific details about the power dynamics, expectations, and desires of each partner. By formalizing the exchange of power, both partners can feel more secure in their roles and committed to the fantasy.

> **Example**
>
> **Scenario 3: The Medical Examination**
> In this scenario, the Dominant takes on the role of a medical professional, conducting a playful examination of the Submissive's "fertility." This roleplay can incorporate elements of medical fetishism, where the Dominant's authority enhances the power exchange. The Submissive may be instructed to respond to the Dominant's commands, heightening the sense of surrender and vulnerability.

Conclusion

Breeding as a power exchange offers a rich tapestry of erotic possibilities, allowing partners to explore their desires within a framework of trust, consent, and communication. By understanding the theoretical foundations and navigating the challenges inherent in this dynamic, couples can create fulfilling and meaningful experiences that deepen their connection and enhance their intimacy. As with any fantasy, the key lies in open dialogue and mutual respect, ensuring that both partners can fully embrace their roles within the breeding narrative.

Roleplaying dominant and submissive breeding dynamics

Roleplaying dominant and submissive breeding dynamics can be an exhilarating exploration of power exchange, intimacy, and fantasy. This section delves into the psychological underpinnings, practical considerations, and creative expressions of this particular kink.

Theoretical Framework

The dynamics of dominance and submission (D/s) are rooted in the interplay of control, trust, and vulnerability. In breeding fantasies, these dynamics can be magnified through the lens of reproductive themes. The dominant partner often embodies the role of the initiator, exerting control over the submissive partner's body and choices, while the submissive partner embraces the vulnerability of their role, which may include the anticipation of conception and the implications of pregnancy.

$$D = f(C, T, V) \qquad (9)$$

Where:

- D = Dominance
- C = Control exerted by the dominant partner
- T = Trust established between partners
- V = Vulnerability experienced by the submissive partner

This equation illustrates that the experience of dominance is a function of control, trust, and vulnerability. A successful breeding fantasy hinges on the balance of these elements, ensuring that both partners feel safe and fulfilled in their roles.

Common Problems and Concerns

While engaging in breeding dynamics, it is crucial to address potential problems that may arise:

- **Consent Issues:** Consent must be explicit and ongoing. Partners should regularly check in with each other to ensure that both are comfortable and willing to continue.

- **Emotional Triggers:** The themes of reproduction and pregnancy can evoke strong emotions. Partners should discuss potential triggers beforehand and establish strategies for managing them.

- **Power Imbalances:** It is vital to recognize and address any power imbalances that may surface. The dominant partner should never exploit their position; instead, they should prioritize the submissive partner's well-being.

- **Societal Stigma:** Engaging in breeding dynamics can attract judgment from outsiders. Partners should prepare for potential societal backlash and develop strategies for dealing with it.

Practical Applications

To effectively roleplay dominant and submissive breeding dynamics, partners can explore various scenarios and techniques:

- **Setting the Scene:** Create an environment that enhances the fantasy. This could include dim lighting, sensual music, or props that signify fertility and reproduction.

- **Character Development:** Each partner can develop their character's backstory, motivations, and desires. This depth can enrich the roleplay experience, making it more immersive.

- **Scripted Scenarios:** Prepare scripts or outlines for specific scenes. For example, the dominant partner may initiate a scenario where they "claim" the submissive partner, emphasizing the breeding aspect.

- **Incorporating Fetish Elements:** Utilize clothing, accessories, or toys that align with the breeding theme. This could include lingerie that accentuates the body, or items that symbolize fertility.

- **Aftercare:** Aftercare is essential in any D/s dynamic, especially in breeding scenarios. Partners should take time to reconnect, discuss feelings, and provide emotional support after the roleplay.

Examples of Roleplay Scenarios

Here are some examples of breeding dynamics that partners can explore:

- **The Fertile Encounter:** The dominant partner emphasizes the submissive's fertility, creating a scenario where they "must" conceive. The dominant partner's assertiveness can heighten the submissive's arousal and sense of vulnerability.

- **The Claiming Ritual:** This scenario involves a ritualistic approach to claiming the submissive partner. The dominant partner may use specific phrases or actions to signify their intention to breed, reinforcing the power dynamic.

- **The Medical Examination:** Incorporating elements of medical play can intensify the experience. The dominant partner could assume the role of a doctor, examining the submissive's reproductive health and discussing the implications of pregnancy.

- **Fantasy of Conception:** Create a scenario where the partners roleplay the act of conception itself, focusing on the physical and emotional sensations involved. This can include verbal affirmations from the dominant partner about the desire to breed.

Conclusion

Roleplaying dominant and submissive breeding dynamics offers a rich terrain for exploration, intimacy, and connection. By understanding the theoretical framework, addressing potential problems, and engaging in practical applications, partners can create a fulfilling and consensual experience. As with all aspects of kink, open communication, trust, and mutual respect are paramount to navigating these fantasies safely and enjoyably.

Through this exploration, partners not only engage in a thrilling fantasy but also deepen their understanding of each other's desires, boundaries, and emotional landscapes, ultimately fostering a more profound connection.

Exploring Breeding Communities and Events

The exploration of breeding communities and events provides a unique lens through which individuals can delve deeper into their breeding fantasies, share experiences, and connect with like-minded individuals. This subsection will discuss the various types of breeding communities, the events associated with them, and the dynamics that characterize these interactions.

Understanding Breeding Communities

Breeding communities are often formed around shared interests in breeding fantasies, pregnancy play, and the associated psychological and physical dynamics. These communities can exist both online and offline, providing spaces for individuals to express their desires without fear of judgment.

Types of Communities Breeding communities can be categorized into several types:

- **Online Forums and Social Media Groups:** Platforms like FetLife, Reddit, and specialized forums allow users to share stories, ask questions, and seek advice on breeding fantasies. These spaces often have threads dedicated to specific interests within the breeding fetish, such as natural conception, artificial insemination, and postpartum roleplay.

- **Local Meetups and Events:** Many cities have local kink and fetish groups that host meetups, workshops, and parties. These events can include discussions on breeding fantasies, roleplay demonstrations, and opportunities for networking with others who share similar interests.

- **Conventions and Festivals:** Larger gatherings, such as BDSM conventions or fetish festivals, often feature panels, workshops, and social events focused on breeding fantasies. These events provide a more immersive experience, allowing participants to engage in roleplay and learn from experts in the field.

The Dynamics of Breeding Events

Participating in breeding events can vary widely in terms of structure and atmosphere. Understanding the dynamics at play can help individuals navigate these experiences more effectively.

Consent and Boundaries At any breeding event, consent is paramount. Participants must engage in clear communication regarding their boundaries and desires. It is essential to establish safewords and protocols for check-ins throughout the event to ensure that all parties feel safe and respected.

Roleplay Scenarios Events may include organized roleplay scenarios where participants can act out their breeding fantasies in a controlled environment. These scenarios can range from light-hearted and playful to more intense and immersive experiences. It is crucial to have a clear understanding of the roles being played and to negotiate the specifics of the scene beforehand.

Emotional Support and Aftercare Aftercare is a vital component of any breeding event. Participants should plan for emotional support following intense roleplay sessions. This can include time spent discussing the experience, checking in on each other's feelings, and engaging in comforting activities to help transition back to everyday life.

Challenges Within Breeding Communities

While breeding communities can provide valuable support and connection, they are not without their challenges.

Stigma and Judgment Participants may face societal stigma surrounding their interests. This can lead to feelings of shame or isolation. It is essential for community members to create inclusive and supportive environments that encourage open dialogue and acceptance.

Power Dynamics Breeding fantasies often involve complex power dynamics, which can lead to misunderstandings or conflicts within communities. It is crucial to address any power imbalances and ensure that all participants are engaging from a place of mutual respect and consent.

Privacy Concerns Given the taboo nature of breeding fantasies, privacy is a significant concern for many participants. Individuals should be mindful of their digital footprint and consider using pseudonyms or anonymous accounts when engaging in online communities. Offline, discretion is equally important; participants should be cautious about sharing personal information.

Examples of Breeding Events and Communities

To illustrate the diversity of breeding communities and events, consider the following examples:

- **The Breeder's Ball:** An annual event that brings together individuals interested in breeding fantasies. The event features workshops on roleplay techniques, discussions on consent, and opportunities for participants to engage in their fantasies in a safe environment.

- **Online Breeding Forums:** Websites dedicated to breeding fantasies where users can share their experiences, seek advice, and connect with others who share similar interests. These forums often have sections for roleplay scenarios, personal stories, and discussions about the psychological aspects of breeding play.

- **Local Kink Meetups:** Many cities host regular kink meetups that include discussions on various fetishes, including breeding. These gatherings provide a space for individuals to share their interests, learn from others, and engage in casual roleplay.

Conclusion

Exploring breeding communities and events can significantly enhance one's understanding of breeding fantasies and provide a supportive network for individuals with similar interests. By prioritizing consent, establishing clear communication, and fostering a sense of community, participants can navigate these spaces safely and enjoyably. As societal perceptions of fetishes and kinks continue to evolve, breeding communities may play a crucial role in normalizing and celebrating these desires, allowing individuals to embrace their fantasies without fear of judgment.

Creating breeding contracts and rituals

Creating breeding contracts and rituals is an essential aspect of engaging in breeding fantasy play. These elements not only enhance the experience but also provide a framework for establishing consent, boundaries, and mutual understanding between partners. In this section, we will explore the theoretical foundations of breeding contracts and rituals, the potential problems that may arise, and practical examples to guide your exploration.

Theoretical Foundations

Breeding contracts and rituals serve multiple purposes in the realm of erotic roleplay. They can be understood through the lens of consensual non-monogamy, BDSM principles, and the psychology of fantasy fulfillment.

1. **Consent and Boundaries**   At the core of any breeding contract is the principle of consent. According to the *Consent Model* (see [?]), all parties involved must agree to the terms of the contract, which should clearly outline what is permissible within

the context of the breeding fantasy. This includes not only the physical acts but also emotional expectations and any potential risks involved.

2. **Psychological Safety** Rituals can create a sense of psychological safety. By engaging in a structured approach to the fantasy, participants can navigate their feelings and desires more effectively. Research indicates that rituals can enhance emotional intimacy and trust (see [?]).

3. **Power Dynamics** Breeding fantasies often involve specific power dynamics, such as dominance and submission. Contracts can delineate these roles, ensuring that both parties are aware of their responsibilities and expectations. This aligns with the *Power Exchange Theory* (see [?]), which emphasizes the importance of clear communication in BDSM dynamics.

Potential Problems

While breeding contracts and rituals can enhance the experience, they may also present challenges. Here are some potential problems to consider:

1. **Miscommunication** One of the most common issues is miscommunication regarding the terms of the contract. If one partner misunderstands the expectations, it can lead to feelings of betrayal or discomfort. To mitigate this risk, it is crucial to engage in open discussions and revisions of the contract as needed.

2. **Emotional Reactions** Engaging in breeding fantasy can evoke strong emotional responses. Participants may find themselves grappling with feelings of jealousy, inadequacy, or fear. It is essential to establish a framework for addressing these emotions, including regular check-ins and aftercare practices.

3. **Changing Dynamics** As relationships evolve, so too may the desires and boundaries of the individuals involved. Contracts should be viewed as living documents that can be revisited and revised as necessary. Failure to adapt to changing dynamics can lead to resentment or conflict.

Practical Examples

To create effective breeding contracts and rituals, consider the following practical examples:

1. Breeding Contract Template   A breeding contract should include the following elements:

- **Parties Involved:** Clearly state the names or pseudonyms of all participants.

- **Purpose:** Define the purpose of the contract, emphasizing the breeding fantasy aspect.

- **Consent:** Include a statement affirming that all parties consent to the terms outlined.

- **Boundaries:** Specify any hard and soft limits, including activities that are off-limits.

- **Communication Protocols:** Outline how participants will communicate during the roleplay, including the use of safewords.

- **Aftercare:** Describe the aftercare practices that will be implemented following the roleplay.

2. Rituals for Engaging in Breeding Fantasy   Rituals can enhance the experience and create a sense of commitment to the fantasy. Here are a few examples:

- **Initiation Ceremony:** Create a special ceremony to mark the beginning of the breeding roleplay. This could involve exchanging tokens or symbols of commitment.

- **Monthly Check-Ins:** Schedule regular check-ins to discuss feelings, desires, and any adjustments needed in the contract. This can be framed as a ritualistic practice to reinforce communication.

- **Celebration of Milestones:** Establish rituals to celebrate milestones within the fantasy, such as the "successful insemination" or reaching a certain stage in the roleplay. This could involve special dates or themed activities.

Conclusion

Creating breeding contracts and rituals is a vital component of engaging in breeding fantasy play. By establishing clear guidelines and incorporating meaningful rituals, participants can enhance their experience, foster emotional intimacy, and navigate the complexities of their desires. As with any aspect of erotic roleplay, open communication, consent, and adaptability are key to ensuring a fulfilling and safe exploration of breeding fantasies.

Breeding fantasies and pregnancy risk awareness

Breeding fantasies often evoke a complex interplay of desire, intimacy, and vulnerability. While these fantasies can be a source of erotic excitement and exploration, it is crucial to approach them with a clear understanding of the associated risks, particularly concerning pregnancy. This section delves into the importance of pregnancy risk awareness within the context of breeding fantasies, highlighting theoretical frameworks, potential problems, and practical examples.

Understanding Pregnancy Risks

Pregnancy, while a natural biological process, carries inherent risks that can vary widely based on individual health, circumstances, and the methods of conception involved. Understanding these risks is essential for anyone engaging in breeding fantasies. The primary risks associated with pregnancy include:

- **Unintended Pregnancy:** Engaging in sexual activities with the intent of conception can lead to unintended pregnancies, which may have profound emotional, social, and financial implications.

- **Health Risks:** Pregnancy can pose health risks to both the pregnant individual and the fetus, including gestational diabetes, preeclampsia, and complications during delivery.

- **Emotional and Psychological Impact:** The emotional landscape surrounding pregnancy can be complex, involving feelings of joy, anxiety, and fear. For some, the prospect of pregnancy can trigger deep-seated issues related to control, body image, and societal expectations.

Theoretical Frameworks

From a psychological perspective, breeding fantasies can be analyzed through various lenses, including:

- **Psychodynamic Theory:** This approach suggests that breeding fantasies may arise from unconscious desires related to fertility, motherhood, and the primal instinct to reproduce. The interplay of these desires can create a powerful erotic charge.

- **Cognitive Behavioral Theory:** This framework posits that individuals may fantasize about breeding as a way to explore their beliefs about sexuality, intimacy, and societal roles. Cognitive distortions, such as catastrophizing the consequences of pregnancy, can influence how these fantasies are experienced.

- **Feminist Theory:** Feminist perspectives emphasize the societal implications of breeding fantasies, particularly regarding gender roles and power dynamics. Understanding these dynamics can help individuals navigate their fantasies with greater awareness of the cultural narratives surrounding reproduction.

Potential Problems and Considerations

Engaging in breeding fantasies without adequate risk awareness can lead to several challenges:

- **Miscommunication:** Partners may have differing views on the desirability of pregnancy, leading to misunderstandings and emotional distress. Clear communication about desires and boundaries is vital.

- **Societal Stigma:** Individuals exploring breeding fantasies may face judgment or stigma from society, which can exacerbate feelings of shame or guilt. It is important to create a safe space for open dialogue about these fantasies.

- **Emotional Triggers:** For some individuals, the theme of pregnancy may trigger past traumas or unresolved issues. Engaging in breeding fantasies requires a thorough understanding of one's emotional landscape and potential triggers.

Practical Examples

To effectively navigate breeding fantasies while maintaining pregnancy risk awareness, individuals can consider the following practical strategies:

- **Open Dialogue:** Partners should engage in candid conversations about their desires, fears, and boundaries related to pregnancy. This dialogue can include discussing the potential for unintended pregnancies and establishing a mutual understanding of consent.

- **Use of Protection:** If the intent is to roleplay breeding scenarios without the actual risk of pregnancy, utilizing appropriate contraception or barriers can help maintain a sense of safety. Discussing the use of condoms or other forms of birth control can be an essential part of the negotiation process.

- **Emotional Check-Ins:** Regular emotional check-ins during roleplay can help partners gauge each other's comfort levels and address any feelings of anxiety or discomfort that may arise. This practice fosters an environment of trust and support.

- **Aftercare:** Engaging in aftercare following breeding roleplay can be crucial for emotional well-being. This may include discussing the experience, providing reassurance, and offering physical comfort to help partners process their feelings.

Conclusion

Breeding fantasies can be a deeply fulfilling aspect of sexual exploration, but they require a careful approach to pregnancy risk awareness. By understanding the potential risks, employing theoretical frameworks to analyze desires, and implementing practical strategies for communication and safety, individuals can navigate these fantasies with greater confidence and emotional security. Ultimately, the goal is to create a space where erotic exploration can coexist with informed consent and mutual respect, allowing for an enriching experience that honors both fantasy and reality.

The importance of aftercare in breeding play

Aftercare is a critical component of any BDSM or kink experience, and it holds particular significance in the context of breeding play. This section explores the multifaceted nature of aftercare, its psychological and emotional benefits, and practical considerations for ensuring a fulfilling and safe experience for all parties involved.

Understanding Aftercare

Aftercare refers to the time and activities that occur after a BDSM scene or roleplay, aimed at helping participants recover emotionally and physically. It is a time for nurturing, reassurance, and reflection, allowing individuals to process their experiences. In breeding play, where themes of vulnerability, power dynamics, and emotional intensity are prevalent, aftercare becomes even more essential.

Psychological Benefits of Aftercare

The psychological impact of breeding play can be profound. Participants may experience a range of emotions, from exhilaration to anxiety, and the transition back to everyday life can be jarring. Aftercare serves several important psychological functions:

- **Emotional Regulation:** Engaging in breeding fantasies can elicit strong feelings, such as joy, fear, or even guilt. Aftercare provides a safe space for individuals to express these emotions and receive support.

- **Reinforcing Trust:** Aftercare is an opportunity to reaffirm the trust established between partners. It demonstrates care and consideration for one another's well-being, fostering a deeper connection.

- **Closure:** Aftercare helps participants process the experience, allowing for closure and reflection. This is particularly important in breeding scenarios, where the themes of conception and pregnancy can evoke complex feelings.

Physical Considerations in Aftercare

In addition to emotional support, aftercare in breeding play may also involve physical care. Participants should consider the following:

- **Hydration and Nutrition:** Engaging in intense roleplay can be physically demanding. Providing water and snacks can help restore energy levels and promote physical well-being.

- **Comfort Measures:** Depending on the nature of the roleplay, participants may need physical comfort, such as cuddling, massage, or simply resting together. This physical closeness can enhance feelings of safety and intimacy.

- **Health Monitoring:** In scenarios involving artificial insemination or medical play, it is crucial to monitor each other's physical health post-scene. Discuss any discomfort or concerns that may arise.

Creating a Personalized Aftercare Plan

Every individual has unique aftercare needs, particularly in the context of breeding play. To create an effective aftercare plan, consider the following steps:

1. **Communicate Preferences:** Before engaging in breeding play, discuss what aftercare looks like for both partners. This may include specific activities, words of affirmation, or physical touch.

2. **Establish Aftercare Rituals:** Develop personalized rituals that signal the end of a scene and transition into aftercare. This could involve specific phrases, gestures, or activities that both partners find comforting.

3. **Check-in Conversations:** After the scene, engage in open conversations about each partner's feelings and experiences. This dialogue can help address any lingering emotions or concerns and deepen the connection.

Addressing Common Problems in Aftercare

Despite the best intentions, aftercare can sometimes present challenges. Here are some common issues and potential solutions:

- **Miscommunication:** Partners may have different expectations for aftercare. To mitigate this, prioritize open dialogue both before and after the scene to clarify needs and preferences.

- **Overwhelming Emotions:** One partner may feel emotionally overwhelmed and struggle to articulate their needs. In such cases, patience and gentle encouragement can help facilitate communication.

- **Physical Discomfort:** If a partner experiences physical discomfort post-scene, it is essential to address this promptly. Discuss any issues and provide appropriate care, such as applying ice or heat, depending on the discomfort.

Examples of Aftercare Activities

Aftercare can take many forms, depending on the preferences of the participants. Here are some examples specifically tailored for breeding play:

- **Cuddling and Skin-to-Skin Contact:** Physical closeness can provide comfort and reassurance, enhancing the emotional bond.

- **Gentle Reassurance:** Verbal affirmations, such as "You did amazing" or "I'm here for you," can help soothe any feelings of insecurity or vulnerability.

- **Reflection Time:** Set aside time to discuss the experience, highlighting what worked well and what could be improved in future sessions.

- **Creating a Safe Space:** Ensure that the environment is calm and inviting, perhaps with soft lighting, comforting blankets, or soothing music to enhance relaxation.

Conclusion

Aftercare is an integral aspect of breeding play, providing essential emotional and physical support to participants. By prioritizing aftercare, individuals can enhance their experiences, deepen their connections, and ensure that all parties feel valued and safe. As with any aspect of kink and BDSM, open communication and mutual understanding are key to creating fulfilling aftercare practices that cater to the unique needs of each participant. Embracing aftercare not only enriches the breeding fantasy but also fosters a culture of care and respect within the kink community.

Safety and Health Considerations

Physical Health

Understanding Reproductive Health

Reproductive health is a critical aspect of overall well-being, encompassing the physical, mental, and social factors that influence an individual's reproductive system and its functions. It is essential to understand reproductive health, particularly in the context of breeding fantasies and erotic pregnancy play, as it informs the choices and practices involved in these experiences.

Defining Reproductive Health

The World Health Organization (WHO) defines reproductive health as a state of complete physical, mental, and social well-being in all matters relating to the reproductive system. This includes the ability to have a satisfying and safe sex life, the capability to reproduce, and the freedom to make informed choices regarding reproduction. It also emphasizes the importance of access to comprehensive reproductive health services, including education, contraception, and maternal care.

Key Components of Reproductive Health

Understanding reproductive health involves recognizing several key components:

- **Menstrual Health:** Regular menstrual cycles are a sign of healthy reproductive function. Menstrual irregularities can indicate underlying health issues, such as polycystic ovary syndrome (PCOS) or hormonal imbalances.

- **Fertility Awareness:** Knowledge of one's fertility cycle is crucial for those interested in conception. This includes understanding ovulation, the fertile window, and methods for tracking fertility, such as basal body temperature charting or ovulation predictor kits.

- **Sexually Transmitted Infections (STIs):** The prevention and treatment of STIs are vital for reproductive health. STIs can have significant implications for fertility and overall health, making regular screenings and safe sex practices essential.

- **Pregnancy Health:** This encompasses preconception care, prenatal care, and postpartum recovery. Understanding the physical and emotional changes during pregnancy is crucial for those engaging in pregnancy play.

- **Contraception:** Access to contraceptive methods allows individuals to plan their reproductive lives. Understanding different contraceptive options and their implications is essential for informed decision-making.

Common Reproductive Health Issues

Several issues can impact reproductive health, and awareness of these can enhance the safety and enjoyment of breeding fantasies:

- **Infertility:** Infertility affects many couples and can be due to various factors, including age, hormonal issues, and lifestyle choices. Understanding the causes of infertility can inform roleplay scenarios that revolve around conception struggles.

- **Pregnancy Complications:** Conditions such as gestational diabetes, preeclampsia, and miscarriage can affect pregnancy. Roleplaying scenarios should consider these factors to maintain a realistic and safe experience.

- **Mental Health:** Emotional well-being is integral to reproductive health. Conditions such as anxiety and depression can influence sexual desire and reproductive choices. Engaging in breeding fantasies may evoke strong emotional responses that require careful navigation.

- **Body Image and Self-Perception:** Many individuals struggle with body image issues, particularly during pregnancy. Understanding these feelings can help partners support each other in roleplay scenarios that involve body modifications or changes associated with pregnancy.

Educating Yourself and Your Partner

Education is a cornerstone of understanding reproductive health. Here are some strategies for enhancing knowledge:

- **Consulting Healthcare Professionals:** Regular check-ups with gynecologists or reproductive health specialists can provide valuable insights into individual reproductive health.

- **Workshops and Classes:** Many organizations offer workshops on reproductive health, fertility awareness, and sexual wellness. Participating in these can deepen understanding and foster open discussions between partners.

- **Researching Reliable Sources:** Accessing reputable sources of information, such as medical journals, books, and websites dedicated to reproductive health, can provide accurate knowledge.

Conclusion

Understanding reproductive health is essential for anyone engaging in breeding fantasies and erotic pregnancy play. By recognizing the physical, emotional, and social dimensions of reproductive health, individuals can create safer, more fulfilling experiences. This knowledge empowers participants to navigate their desires while prioritizing health and well-being.

Incorporating this understanding into roleplay scenarios not only enhances the erotic experience but also fosters a deeper connection and trust between partners. As you explore breeding fantasies, remember that informed consent and mutual respect are paramount, ensuring that all experiences are enjoyable and safe for everyone involved.

Safe practices for roleplaying pregnancy

Roleplaying pregnancy can be an exhilarating exploration of fantasies and desires, but it is essential to prioritize safety and health throughout the experience. Engaging in this type of roleplay requires careful consideration of both physical and emotional well-being. This section outlines safe practices to ensure that participants can fully enjoy their fantasies while minimizing risks.

Understanding the Risks

Before delving into specific practices, it is crucial to recognize the potential risks associated with pregnancy roleplay. These may include:

- **Physical Health Risks:** Engaging in activities that mimic pregnancy can lead to physical discomfort or strain, particularly if props or costumes are involved. Additionally, if roleplay includes sexual activity, there are inherent risks of sexually transmitted infections (STIs) and unintended pregnancies.

- **Emotional Risks:** Pregnancy can evoke a wide range of emotions, from joy to anxiety. Roleplaying scenarios that touch on sensitive topics, such as infertility or pregnancy loss, may trigger emotional responses that require careful handling.

- **Social Risks:** Engaging in public displays of pregnancy roleplay can attract attention and judgment from others, which may lead to feelings of shame or embarrassment.

Setting Clear Boundaries

Establishing clear boundaries is vital for ensuring that all participants feel safe and respected. This involves:

- **Pre-Roleplay Discussions:** Before engaging in any roleplay, partners should have open discussions about their desires, limits, and any specific scenarios they wish to explore. This conversation should include topics such as:
    - What aspects of pregnancy are appealing?
    - Are there any hard limits (e.g., no discussions of loss or medical complications)?
    - What are the preferred methods of communication during the roleplay?

- **Establishing Safewords:** Safewords are essential for maintaining a safe environment. Participants should agree on a word or signal that can be used to pause or stop the roleplay if it becomes uncomfortable or triggering.

Physical Safety Practices

When roleplaying pregnancy, physical safety should be a top priority. Here are several practices to consider:

PHYSICAL HEALTH 125

- **Use of Props:** If using props such as pregnancy bellies or costumes, ensure they are comfortable and do not restrict movement or breathing. For example, inflatable pregnancy bellies can be a fun addition, but they should be securely fastened and checked for any potential hazards.

- **Positioning and Movement:** Be mindful of physical positions that may strain the body. Pregnant individuals often experience discomfort in certain positions, so it is important to choose scenarios that allow for comfort and mobility. Consider using soft cushions or pillows to support the body during roleplay.

- **Hygiene Practices:** If sexual activity is involved, ensure that safe sex practices are in place. This includes using condoms to prevent STIs and unintended pregnancies. Additionally, maintain cleanliness with props and costumes to avoid infections.

Emotional Safety Practices

Emotional safety is just as important as physical safety. Here are strategies to support emotional well-being during pregnancy roleplay:

- **Aftercare:** Aftercare is an essential component of any roleplay, particularly one as emotionally charged as pregnancy. Aftercare can include cuddling, discussing the experience, and providing reassurance. This helps participants process their feelings and reinforces the bond between partners.

- **Check-Ins:** Regular check-ins during the roleplay can help gauge comfort levels. Simple questions such as "How are you feeling?" or "Do you want to continue?" can provide an opportunity for participants to express any discomfort or desire to change the scenario.

- **Preparation for Emotional Triggers:** Be aware of potential emotional triggers that may arise during the roleplay. Discuss these in advance and have a plan for how to handle them. For instance, if one partner has experienced pregnancy loss, it may be beneficial to avoid scenarios that evoke those feelings.

Handling Social Risks

Engaging in pregnancy roleplay can attract attention, especially if it occurs in public settings. Here are some practices to mitigate social risks:

- **Choosing the Right Environment:** Consider the setting for roleplay. Private spaces, such as home or designated kink-friendly locations, can provide a safer environment compared to public spaces where onlookers may not understand the context.

- **Discretion in Public:** If roleplaying in public, maintain discretion to avoid unwanted attention. This may involve subtlety in costumes or behaviors that signal the roleplay without being overtly provocative.

- **Educating Others:** If comfortable, educate friends or family about your interests in pregnancy roleplay. This can help reduce stigma and create a supportive environment for your exploration.

Conclusion

In conclusion, safe practices for roleplaying pregnancy involve a multifaceted approach that prioritizes physical and emotional well-being. By establishing clear boundaries, utilizing safe props, and maintaining open communication, participants can enjoy their fantasies while minimizing risks. Ultimately, the goal is to create an enriching and pleasurable experience that respects the desires and limits of all involved.

$$\text{Safety} = \text{Communication} + \text{Consent} + \text{Aftercare} \qquad (10)$$

STI and Pregnancy Risk Prevention

In the realm of breeding fantasy and erotic pregnancy play, understanding and mitigating the risks associated with sexually transmitted infections (STIs) and unintended pregnancies is paramount. This section delves into the necessary precautions, safe practices, and educational insights to ensure a fulfilling experience while prioritizing health and safety.

Understanding STIs

Sexually transmitted infections are infections that are primarily spread through sexual contact. Common STIs include chlamydia, gonorrhea, syphilis, herpes, human immunodeficiency virus (HIV), and human papillomavirus (HPV). Each of these infections can have significant implications for reproductive health, particularly in the context of pregnancy.

PHYSICAL HEALTH 127

Risks Associated with STIs

The presence of STIs can lead to various complications during pregnancy, including:

- **Preterm Labor:** Infections can trigger early labor, leading to preterm birth, which poses health risks for the newborn.

- **Low Birth Weight:** STIs can contribute to low birth weight, increasing the likelihood of health issues for the infant.

- **Transmission to the Baby:** Certain STIs can be transmitted from mother to child during childbirth, potentially causing serious health problems.

- **Infertility:** Untreated STIs can lead to pelvic inflammatory disease (PID), which may result in infertility or ectopic pregnancies.

Prevention Strategies

To minimize the risks associated with STIs and unintended pregnancies, individuals engaging in breeding fantasy should adopt the following prevention strategies:

1. Communication and Testing Open communication with partners about sexual health is essential. Regular STI testing for all partners can help identify infections early and reduce the risk of transmission. It is advisable to establish a testing routine, particularly before engaging in any new sexual relationship or roleplay scenario.

2. Safe Sex Practices Utilizing barrier methods, such as condoms or dental dams, can significantly reduce the risk of STI transmission. While these methods may not fully align with the fantasy of breeding, they can be essential in protecting against infections. Discussing the use of barriers within the context of roleplay can enhance safety without detracting from the experience.

3. Vaccinations Vaccinations are available for certain STIs, such as HPV and hepatitis B. Staying up-to-date with vaccinations can provide an additional layer of protection against infections that can impact reproductive health.

4. Understanding Fertility Awareness Engaging in fertility awareness methods can help individuals understand their reproductive cycles, including ovulation periods. This understanding can aid in timing sexual activity for conception while also enabling individuals to navigate the risks associated with unintended pregnancies.

The Role of Consent and Boundaries

In any roleplay scenario involving breeding fantasy, consent remains a cornerstone of safety. Establishing clear boundaries regarding sexual health and the potential for pregnancy is crucial. Partners should engage in open discussions about their desires, fears, and health status, ensuring that all parties feel comfortable and respected.

Example Scenarios

Consider the following scenarios that illustrate the importance of STI and pregnancy risk prevention in breeding fantasy:

Scenario 1: The Trusting Couple   A couple engages in breeding fantasy roleplay, discussing their desire to explore natural conception. Before proceeding, they agree to undergo STI testing and share their results. They also decide to use condoms during initial encounters to ensure safety while gradually increasing intimacy as trust builds.

Scenario 2: The Fantasy with Safeguards   In another scenario, a couple wishes to incorporate elements of artificial insemination into their roleplay. They discuss using a sterile syringe for insemination while employing barrier methods to prevent STIs. They establish a safeword to pause the roleplay if either partner feels uncomfortable or anxious about health risks.

Conclusion

Understanding STI and pregnancy risk prevention is essential for anyone engaging in breeding fantasy and erotic pregnancy play. By prioritizing open communication, regular testing, safe sex practices, and informed consent, individuals can create a safe and pleasurable environment for exploration. Emphasizing health and safety does not detract from the experience; rather, it enhances the intimacy and trust that are foundational to fulfilling sexual encounters.

Pregnancy fetish and body modifications

The intersection of pregnancy fetish and body modifications represents a fascinating realm within eroticism, where the physicality of the body is both celebrated and transformed to enhance the allure of pregnancy. This section explores the motivations behind body modifications related to pregnancy fantasies, the psychological implications, and the challenges that arise from such practices.

Understanding Pregnancy Fetishism

Pregnancy fetishism, often referred to as "pregnancy kink," involves a sexual attraction to the state of pregnancy. This attraction can manifest in various ways, including a fascination with the physical changes that accompany pregnancy, such as a growing belly, increased breast size, and the overall nurturing aura associated with expectant mothers. The allure of pregnancy can be tied to themes of fertility, femininity, and the primal aspects of human reproduction.

Body Modifications in Pregnancy Fantasy

Body modifications, in the context of pregnancy fetishism, can range from temporary enhancements to more permanent alterations. Common forms of body modifications that align with pregnancy fantasies include:

- **Prosthetic Bellies:** Many individuals interested in pregnancy play opt for prosthetic bellies that simulate the appearance of pregnancy. These prosthetics can vary in size and shape, allowing participants to embody different stages of pregnancy. The psychological impact of wearing a prosthetic belly can enhance the roleplay experience, creating a deeper connection to the fantasy.

- **Breast Augmentation:** Some may seek breast augmentation to achieve a fuller, more voluptuous appearance, which is often associated with pregnancy. This modification can serve to enhance the physical attributes that are typically celebrated in pregnancy fetishism.

- **Tummy Tattoos and Art:** Temporary tattoos or body art that celebrates pregnancy themes can be used to adorn the belly. This practice not only personalizes the experience but also allows for creative expression within the context of the fantasy.

- **Weight Gain:** Some individuals may engage in controlled weight gain to mimic the physical changes of pregnancy. This can be a complex and sensitive area, as it may intersect with issues of body image and self-esteem.

- **Medical Play:** Incorporating elements of medical play, such as the use of medical devices or props that signify pregnancy, can enhance the experience. This may include items like ultrasound machines or pregnancy tests, which can add a layer of realism to the roleplay.

Psychological Implications

The motivations behind body modifications in pregnancy fetishism can be multifaceted. For some, these modifications serve as a means of embodying their fantasies, allowing them to explore their desires in a tangible way. The act of altering one's body can also provide a sense of empowerment, as individuals take control of their physical appearance to align with their erotic fantasies.

However, it is crucial to recognize the psychological challenges that may accompany body modifications. Issues of body image, societal pressure, and the potential for negative self-perception can arise. It is essential for individuals engaging in body modifications to maintain a strong sense of self-awareness and to prioritize mental health throughout their journey.

Ethical Considerations

Engaging in body modifications for the sake of pregnancy fetishism also raises ethical considerations. It is paramount to approach these practices with an understanding of consent, safety, and the potential impact on relationships. Open communication with partners about desires, boundaries, and the motivations behind body modifications can foster a healthier exploration of pregnancy fantasies.

Conclusion

The interplay between pregnancy fetishism and body modifications offers a rich landscape for exploration and self-discovery. By understanding the motivations, challenges, and ethical considerations surrounding these practices, individuals can navigate their desires in a way that is both fulfilling and respectful. As society continues to evolve in its understanding of sexuality and body autonomy, the dialogue surrounding pregnancy fetishism and body modifications will undoubtedly expand, paving the way for more inclusive and accepting spaces for exploration.

Dealing with physical discomfort during roleplay

Engaging in breeding fantasy and erotic pregnancy play can evoke a myriad of physical sensations, some pleasurable and others potentially uncomfortable. Understanding how to manage physical discomfort during roleplay is essential to ensure a safe, enjoyable, and consensual experience. This section will explore common sources of discomfort, strategies for alleviation, and the importance of communication and aftercare.

Common Sources of Discomfort

Physical discomfort during breeding roleplay can arise from several factors, including:

- **Positioning and Physical Strain:** Certain roleplay scenarios may require specific positions that could lead to strain or discomfort. For example, prolonged kneeling or lying in an awkward position can cause muscle fatigue or joint pain.

- **Costumes and Props:** The use of costumes, such as tight clothing or pregnancy simulation suits, can create discomfort. Materials that do not breathe well or are too restrictive can lead to overheating or skin irritation.

- **Physical Sensations:** The psychological aspects of pregnancy play may trigger physical sensations that mimic discomfort associated with pregnancy, such as bloating or pressure in the abdomen, which can be distressing if not anticipated.

- **Emotional Responses:** Engaging in roleplay that touches on sensitive topics—such as fertility struggles or pregnancy loss—can elicit emotional discomfort that manifests physically, such as tension headaches or stomachaches.

Strategies for Alleviation

To mitigate physical discomfort during roleplay, participants should consider the following strategies:

1. **Preparation and Warm-Up:** Prior to engaging in roleplay, participants should engage in light stretching or warm-up exercises to prepare their bodies for physical activity. This can help prevent strain and increase flexibility.

2. **Setting Boundaries:** Establish clear boundaries regarding what is comfortable and what is not. This includes discussing any pre-existing conditions that may affect physical comfort, such as back pain or joint issues.

3. **Choosing Appropriate Attire:** Select costumes and props that allow for movement and comfort. Fabrics should be breathable, and clothing should not be overly tight. Consider using adjustable or elastic materials that can accommodate different body types and movements.

4. **Regular Check-Ins:** During the roleplay, participants should engage in regular check-ins to assess comfort levels. Simple questions like, "Are you okay?" or "Do you need a break?" can facilitate open communication and address discomfort before it escalates.

5. **Utilizing Props Mindfully:** When using props, ensure they are safe and designed for the intended use. For instance, if using a pregnancy simulation belly, ensure it is not too heavy or restrictive. Consider using lighter alternatives or adjusting the way it is worn.

6. **Aftercare:** Aftercare is crucial for addressing any physical discomfort experienced during the roleplay. This can include physical comfort measures such as massages, providing hydration, or using heat packs on sore areas. Emotional support through discussion and reassurance is equally important.

The Role of Communication

Effective communication is paramount in managing discomfort. Participants should feel empowered to express their needs and concerns without fear of judgment. A collaborative approach to discomfort ensures that both partners can enjoy the experience fully.

$$\text{Comfort Level} = \text{Communication} + \text{Trust} + \text{Consent} \qquad (11)$$

This equation highlights that comfort during roleplay is directly proportional to the quality of communication, the level of trust established, and the clarity of consent between partners.

Conclusion

Dealing with physical discomfort during breeding fantasy and erotic pregnancy play is a multifaceted endeavor that requires awareness, preparation, and open communication. By recognizing potential sources of discomfort and employing strategies for alleviation, participants can create a more enjoyable and fulfilling experience. Aftercare and ongoing dialogue are essential components that not only address immediate discomfort but also foster a deeper connection between partners, enhancing the overall intimacy of the roleplay.

Pregnancy-related health concerns

Pregnancy is a complex physiological state that brings about a myriad of changes in a woman's body. Understanding these changes is crucial, especially in the context of erotic pregnancy play, where the fantasy may intersect with real-life health concerns. This section will explore various pregnancy-related health issues that may arise during roleplay scenarios, emphasizing the need for awareness, safety, and communication.

Common Pregnancy-Related Health Issues

1. **Gestational Diabetes:** This condition occurs when a woman develops high blood sugar levels during pregnancy. It typically arises in the second or third trimester and may require dietary changes, monitoring of blood sugar levels, and sometimes insulin therapy. Roleplayers should be aware of this condition, as it can affect the physical well-being of the person embodying pregnancy in their scenarios.

$$\text{Blood Sugar Level} = \frac{\text{Glucose (mg/dL)}}{\text{Plasma Volume (L)}} \qquad (12)$$

2. **Hypertension:** High blood pressure can develop during pregnancy, leading to conditions like preeclampsia. This condition is characterized by high blood pressure and signs of damage to another organ system, often the kidneys. Symptoms include severe headaches, vision changes, and upper abdominal pain. Participants in pregnancy roleplay should be mindful of these symptoms and prioritize health and safety.

3. **Nausea and Vomiting (Morning Sickness):** Many pregnant individuals experience nausea and vomiting, particularly in the first trimester. While often a normal part of pregnancy, severe cases can lead to dehydration and require medical intervention. Roleplay scenarios should consider the potential for discomfort and the need for breaks or adjustments to maintain a safe and enjoyable experience.

4. **Physical Discomfort:** As the body changes, individuals may experience back pain, pelvic pressure, and joint discomfort. These physical challenges can impact the ability to engage in certain roleplay activities. It is essential to discuss these discomforts openly and to adapt scenarios to accommodate them.

5. **Infections:** Pregnant individuals are at a higher risk for certain infections, including urinary tract infections (UTIs) and sexually transmitted infections (STIs). The physiological changes during pregnancy can alter the immune response, making it vital for participants to discuss and practice safe sex, even within roleplay contexts.

Mental Health Considerations

Pregnancy can also have significant psychological effects. Roleplay scenarios that involve pregnancy should consider the emotional well-being of all participants.

1. **Anxiety and Depression:** The hormonal changes that occur during pregnancy can lead to mood swings and increased anxiety. Participants should be sensitive to these potential emotional shifts and should establish a supportive environment.

2. **Body Image Issues:** Changes in body shape and size can lead to body image concerns. Roleplayers should engage in open dialogue about body positivity and the emotional aspects of embodying pregnancy.

3. **Postpartum Mental Health:** After giving birth, individuals may experience postpartum depression or anxiety. This can impact the dynamics of roleplay if the scenario extends into the postpartum phase. Understanding the emotional complexities of this period is crucial for maintaining a safe and consensual environment.

Communication and Consent

Given the potential health concerns associated with pregnancy, clear communication and consent are paramount. Participants should engage in discussions about their health histories, any existing conditions, and how these may impact their roleplay experiences.

1. **Establishing Health Protocols:** Before engaging in pregnancy roleplay, it is advisable to create a health protocol that outlines what is acceptable and what precautions should be taken. This can include discussing any medical conditions, medications, or lifestyle factors that could influence the roleplay.

2. **Regular Check-ins:** During roleplay, participants should conduct regular check-ins to ensure that everyone is comfortable and safe. This can help address any emerging health concerns promptly and maintain an open dialogue about physical and emotional states.

3. **Aftercare:** Aftercare is an essential component of any roleplay, particularly those involving intense emotional or physical experiences. Participants should prioritize aftercare to address any health concerns and support each other emotionally after a session.

Conclusion

Incorporating pregnancy-related health considerations into erotic roleplay scenarios enriches the experience while ensuring safety and consent. By understanding the

PHYSICAL HEALTH 135

potential health issues that may arise, participants can create a more informed and pleasurable environment. Open communication, mutual respect, and a commitment to health and safety are vital components of integrating these fantasies into one's intimate life.

Sharing fantasies with medical professionals

Engaging with medical professionals about personal fantasies, particularly those related to breeding and pregnancy play, can be a complex and sensitive topic. It is essential to approach these conversations with care, ensuring that both parties feel comfortable and respected. This section explores the theoretical foundations, potential challenges, and practical examples of discussing such intimate subjects with healthcare providers.

Theoretical Foundations

The intersection of sexuality and healthcare has been a subject of interest within the fields of psychology and sexology. Theories such as the *Kinsey Scale* and *Masters and Johnson's Human Sexual Response Cycle* highlight the spectrum of human sexuality and the importance of understanding individual desires. According to Kinsey, sexual orientation and preferences exist on a continuum, which implies that fantasies, including breeding fantasies, can be a normal part of human sexuality.

Moreover, the *Health Belief Model* suggests that individuals are more likely to engage in health-promoting behaviors if they believe they are at risk for a health problem and perceive the benefits of taking action. This model can be applied when discussing fantasies with medical professionals, as individuals may seek reassurance about their sexual health and well-being.

Challenges in Communication

1. **Fear of Judgment**: One of the primary barriers to sharing fantasies with medical professionals is the fear of being judged or misunderstood. Many individuals worry that their fantasies may be deemed abnormal or pathological. This fear can lead to avoidance of open communication, which is crucial for comprehensive healthcare.

2. **Lack of Understanding**: Medical professionals may not always be well-versed in the nuances of sexual fantasies, particularly those that fall outside conventional norms. This lack of understanding can result in inadequate responses

or dismissive attitudes, further discouraging patients from sharing their experiences.

3. **Confidentiality Concerns**: Patients may also worry about the confidentiality of their discussions, fearing that their personal information could be disclosed or that they could be stigmatized within the medical community.

4. **Power Dynamics**: The inherent power dynamics in the doctor-patient relationship can complicate discussions about sexual fantasies. Patients may feel vulnerable and may struggle to assert their needs or desires in the face of perceived authority.

Practical Examples

To facilitate open communication, consider the following strategies when sharing breeding fantasies with medical professionals:

1. **Choose the Right Provider**: Seek out healthcare professionals who are known for their openness to discussing sexual health and desires. This could include sex therapists, gynecologists with a focus on sexual health, or general practitioners with a reputation for being non-judgmental.

2. **Prepare for the Conversation**: Before the appointment, take some time to reflect on what you want to discuss. Writing down your thoughts can help clarify your feelings and make it easier to articulate your desires during the consultation.

3. **Use Clear Language**: When discussing your fantasies, use clear and direct language. For example, you might say, "I have a fantasy about pregnancy that I'd like to explore in a safe and healthy way. Can we discuss any potential health implications?"

4. **Frame It Within Health Context**: Position your fantasy within the context of your overall sexual health. You might say, "I'm interested in understanding how my fantasies about breeding could impact my reproductive health and what precautions I should take."

5. **Ask Open-Ended Questions**: Encourage dialogue by asking open-ended questions. For instance, "How can I safely explore my interests while maintaining my health?" This approach invites the professional to engage with you in a more meaningful way.

6. **Seek Supportive Resources**: If you encounter resistance or discomfort in discussing your fantasies, consider seeking out supportive resources such as sex therapy or sexual health workshops. These environments can provide a more accepting space for exploring your desires.

Conclusion

Sharing breeding fantasies with medical professionals is an essential aspect of maintaining sexual health and well-being. By understanding the theoretical frameworks surrounding sexuality, recognizing potential communication challenges, and employing practical strategies, individuals can foster open and productive discussions with their healthcare providers. Ultimately, these conversations can lead to a more nuanced understanding of one's sexual health, paving the way for a fulfilling and safe exploration of personal fantasies.

Post-pregnancy recovery and self-care

Post-pregnancy recovery is a multifaceted process that encompasses physical, emotional, and psychological dimensions. Engaging in self-care during this period is crucial for individuals who have experienced pregnancy play, whether in fantasy or reality. This section explores the various aspects of post-pregnancy recovery and self-care, emphasizing the importance of holistic approaches to well-being.

Physical Recovery

The physical recovery process after pregnancy, whether real or roleplayed, can be demanding. It involves several physiological changes, including hormonal fluctuations, changes in body shape, and potential physical discomfort. Recognizing these changes is essential for effective self-care.

Hormonal Fluctuations Following pregnancy, the body undergoes significant hormonal shifts. These changes can affect mood, energy levels, and physical health. For example, a decrease in progesterone and estrogen levels can lead to feelings of fatigue and emotional instability. Understanding these hormonal changes can help individuals anticipate and manage their emotional responses.

Body Shape and Physical Discomfort Post-pregnancy, individuals may experience changes in body shape and size. This can lead to feelings of insecurity or dissatisfaction with one's body. Engaging in body-positive practices, such as affirmations and mindful movement, can aid in fostering a healthy relationship with one's body. For instance, gentle exercises like yoga or walking can promote physical recovery while enhancing body awareness.

Emotional Well-being

Emotional recovery is equally important and can be influenced by the dynamics of roleplay and fantasy. Individuals may experience a range of emotions, including joy, anxiety, and even grief related to the end of a roleplaying scenario.

Processing Emotions It is vital to create a space for processing emotions that arise post-pregnancy. Journaling can be an effective tool for self-reflection, allowing individuals to articulate their feelings about the experience. For example, writing about the excitement of the roleplay, the intimacy shared, or even any feelings of loss can provide clarity and emotional relief.

Seeking Support Emotional support from partners, friends, or online communities can significantly enhance recovery. Engaging in discussions about experiences, sharing feelings, and seeking advice can foster a sense of belonging and understanding. Additionally, professional support from therapists specializing in sexual health or postpartum care can be beneficial for navigating complex emotions.

Psychological Aspects

The psychological impact of pregnancy play can extend beyond the immediate experience. It is essential to address any psychological challenges that may arise during recovery.

Fantasy vs. Reality Post-pregnancy, individuals may grapple with the distinction between fantasy and reality. This can lead to feelings of confusion or guilt. It is crucial to engage in self-compassion and recognize that exploring fantasies is a normal part of human sexuality. Creating a clear boundary between fantasy and reality can help in managing expectations and emotional responses.

Addressing Guilt and Shame Feelings of guilt or shame may emerge, particularly if societal norms or personal beliefs conflict with one's desires. Engaging in open conversations about these feelings, whether with a partner or a therapist, can aid in reframing these emotions. Understanding that fantasies do not dictate one's moral character can alleviate feelings of shame.

Practical Self-care Strategies

Implementing practical self-care strategies can promote recovery and enhance overall well-being. Here are some effective approaches:

Physical Self-Care   1. **Nutrition:** Eating a balanced diet rich in vitamins and minerals can support physical recovery. Foods high in iron, calcium, and omega-3 fatty acids are particularly beneficial. 2. **Hydration:** Staying hydrated is vital for physical health. Drinking adequate water can help with energy levels and bodily functions. 3. **Rest:** Prioritizing rest is crucial. Engaging in restorative practices, such as napping or meditative breathing, can help recharge both physically and emotionally.

Emotional Self-care   1. **Mindfulness and Meditation:** Practicing mindfulness can help in grounding oneself and managing anxiety. Techniques such as deep breathing or guided meditations can be beneficial. 2. **Creative Outlets:** Engaging in creative activities, such as painting, writing, or crafting, can provide an emotional release and foster self-expression. 3. **Community Engagement:** Participating in community events or support groups can provide a sense of belonging and reduce feelings of isolation.

Conclusion

In conclusion, post-pregnancy recovery and self-care are essential components of the overall experience of pregnancy play. By acknowledging the physical, emotional, and psychological aspects of recovery, individuals can cultivate a holistic approach to self-care. Emphasizing the importance of support, self-compassion, and practical strategies can empower individuals to navigate this complex journey with grace and confidence. Ultimately, embracing self-care not only enhances recovery but also enriches the experience of exploring one's desires and fantasies in a safe and fulfilling manner.

Mental and Emotional Well-being

Emotional challenges of pregnancy play

Engaging in pregnancy play can evoke a complex array of emotions, both positive and negative. Understanding these emotional challenges is crucial for participants to navigate their fantasies safely and healthily. This section delves into the psychological landscape of pregnancy roleplay, highlighting potential issues and offering insights into managing these emotional dynamics.

1. The Duality of Desire and Fear

Pregnancy fantasies often embody a duality where desire and fear coexist. On one hand, the allure of creating life can be intensely erotic, tapping into deep-seated desires for intimacy, connection, and the primal instincts associated with reproduction. On the other hand, the fear of unwanted consequences, such as actual pregnancy, societal judgment, and personal inadequacies, can loom large.

Example: A participant may fantasize about the thrill of conception, but simultaneously grapple with anxiety over the implications of pregnancy. This tension can lead to internal conflict, where the desire to engage in the fantasy is overshadowed by the fear of its reality. This paradox can manifest as guilt or shame, particularly for those who feel societal pressure to conform to traditional views on pregnancy and motherhood.

2. The Impact of Past Experiences

Individual histories significantly influence how participants engage with pregnancy play. Past experiences with pregnancy, whether positive or negative, can shape emotional responses. For instance, someone who has experienced pregnancy loss may find certain aspects of pregnancy roleplay triggering.

Theory: According to attachment theory, individuals develop emotional responses based on early interactions and relationships. Those with insecure attachment styles may experience heightened anxiety during roleplay scenarios, fearing abandonment or rejection.

Example: A participant who has faced infertility struggles may feel a mix of longing and despair when engaging in breeding fantasies. The fantasy may serve as a coping mechanism, yet it can also amplify feelings of inadequacy or loss. Recognizing these triggers is vital for maintaining emotional safety.

3. Navigating Societal Stigmas

Societal attitudes towards pregnancy and sexuality can create additional emotional hurdles. The stigma surrounding non-traditional sexual fantasies can lead to feelings

MENTAL AND EMOTIONAL WELL-BEING

of isolation or shame. Participants may fear judgment from peers, family, or society at large, which can inhibit open communication about their desires.

Example: A couple interested in exploring breeding fantasies may hesitate to discuss their interests with friends or family, fearing negative reactions. This secrecy can breed feelings of loneliness and shame, complicating the emotional landscape of their relationship.

4. Managing Emotional Triggers

Recognizing and managing emotional triggers is essential for participants in pregnancy play. This involves establishing clear communication and understanding each other's emotional landscapes. Setting boundaries and creating a safe space for dialogue can help mitigate the impact of triggering situations.

Strategies:

- **Pre-Roleplay Check-Ins:** Prior to engaging in pregnancy roleplay, partners should conduct check-ins to discuss feelings, boundaries, and potential triggers. This proactive approach fosters a sense of safety and openness.

- **Post-Roleplay Debriefing:** After the roleplay, participants should engage in a debriefing session to discuss their emotional experiences. This practice can help process feelings and reinforce emotional connection.

5. The Importance of Aftercare

Aftercare is a critical component of any roleplay scenario, particularly in emotionally charged contexts like pregnancy play. Aftercare involves providing emotional support and reassurance following the roleplay, helping participants transition back to their everyday selves.

Example: After an intense session of pregnancy roleplay, one partner may need reassurance and physical comfort, such as cuddling or verbal affirmations. This aftercare can help mitigate any emotional fallout and reinforce trust within the relationship.

6. Seeking Professional Support

For some individuals, the emotional challenges associated with pregnancy play may require professional intervention. Engaging with a therapist who specializes in sexual health or kink-aware therapy can provide valuable insights and coping strategies.

Theory: Cognitive Behavioral Therapy (CBT) can be particularly effective in addressing anxiety and guilt related to sexual fantasies. By reframing negative thoughts and beliefs, individuals can develop healthier perspectives on their desires.

Example: A person struggling with feelings of guilt over their breeding fantasy may benefit from CBT techniques that challenge and reframe these beliefs, promoting self-acceptance and understanding.

7. Conclusion

Emotional challenges in pregnancy play are multifaceted and deeply personal. By acknowledging the complexities of desire, fear, societal stigma, and individual experiences, participants can create a more enriching and supportive environment for exploration. Open communication, boundary-setting, and aftercare are essential tools for navigating these emotional landscapes, allowing individuals to engage in their fantasies with confidence and emotional safety. Ultimately, understanding and addressing these challenges can lead to deeper intimacy and connection within the context of breeding fantasies.

Dealing with emotional triggers

Emotional triggers can significantly impact the experience of those engaging in breeding fantasies and erotic pregnancy play. Understanding and managing these triggers is crucial for maintaining a safe, consensual, and enjoyable environment. This section explores the nature of emotional triggers, their origins, and strategies for effectively dealing with them.

Understanding Emotional Triggers

Emotional triggers are stimuli that provoke strong emotional responses, often linked to past experiences, traumas, or unresolved feelings. In the context of breeding fantasy, triggers may arise from:

MENTAL AND EMOTIONAL WELL-BEING

- **Personal History:** Previous experiences with pregnancy, loss, or fertility issues can evoke powerful emotions during roleplay.

- **Societal Pressures:** Cultural narratives surrounding motherhood and fertility can create stress and anxiety, particularly for those who may feel societal expectations weighing upon them.

- **Relationship Dynamics:** The dynamics between partners, including power imbalances or unresolved conflicts, can contribute to emotional responses during play.

Theoretical Framework

The psychological understanding of emotional triggers can be framed within several theories:

- **Attachment Theory:** This theory posits that early relationships with caregivers shape emotional responses and coping mechanisms in adulthood. Individuals with insecure attachment styles may be more prone to heightened emotional reactions during intimate scenarios.

- **Cognitive Behavioral Theory (CBT):** CBT suggests that thoughts, feelings, and behaviors are interconnected. Identifying negative thought patterns related to pregnancy or intimacy can help individuals manage their emotional triggers.

- **Trauma-Informed Care:** This approach emphasizes understanding the impact of trauma on individuals' lives. Recognizing triggers as potential responses to past trauma can foster empathy and support within relationships.

Identifying Triggers

Recognizing personal triggers is the first step in managing them. This can involve:

1. **Self-Reflection:** Journaling about feelings and experiences related to breeding fantasies can help identify patterns and triggers.

2. **Open Communication:** Discussing feelings with partners can create a supportive environment where both parties feel safe to express concerns and fears.

3. **Therapeutic Support:** Seeking therapy or counseling can provide additional tools for understanding and managing emotional triggers.

Strategies for Managing Triggers

Once triggers are identified, several strategies can be employed to manage them effectively:

- **Establishing Safe Words:** Safe words are essential in any BDSM or roleplay scenario. They allow participants to communicate discomfort without breaking the flow of play. Establishing a safe word that signals a need to pause or stop can help manage overwhelming emotions.

- **Setting Boundaries:** Clearly defining what is off-limits during roleplay can help mitigate the risk of triggering experiences. This includes discussing specific topics or scenarios that may evoke strong emotional responses.

- **Implementing Check-Ins:** Regularly checking in with each other during roleplay can help gauge comfort levels and emotional states. This practice fosters open communication and allows for adjustments as needed.

- **Practicing Mindfulness:** Mindfulness techniques, such as deep breathing or grounding exercises, can help individuals stay present and manage anxiety when faced with emotional triggers.

Aftercare and Emotional Support

Aftercare is a critical component of any intimate or roleplay experience, particularly when emotional triggers are involved. It provides an opportunity for partners to reconnect, process their experiences, and offer emotional support. Aftercare can include:

- **Physical Comfort:** Cuddling, holding hands, or providing a safe space to unwind can help soothe emotional distress.

- **Verbal Reassurance:** Sharing affirmations and discussing positive aspects of the experience can help alleviate any lingering discomfort.

- **Debriefing:** Engaging in a conversation about what worked, what didn't, and how each partner felt during the roleplay can foster understanding and strengthen the relationship.

Conclusion

Dealing with emotional triggers in breeding fantasies and erotic pregnancy play requires awareness, communication, and a commitment to creating a safe space for exploration. By understanding the origins of triggers, employing effective management strategies, and prioritizing aftercare, partners can navigate the complexities of these fantasies with care and intimacy. Ultimately, the goal is to foster an environment where both partners feel empowered to explore their desires while respecting their emotional boundaries.

Roleplaying pregnancy loss and grief

Roleplaying pregnancy loss and grief is a delicate and profound aspect of breeding fantasy that requires sensitivity, understanding, and careful negotiation between partners. This section explores the emotional landscape of pregnancy loss roleplay, the psychological implications involved, and practical considerations for engaging in this type of play.

Understanding the Emotional Landscape

Pregnancy loss can encompass a variety of experiences, including miscarriage, stillbirth, and the loss of a newborn. Each of these experiences carries its own set of emotions, such as grief, guilt, anger, and confusion. Roleplaying these scenarios can serve as a means of exploring complex emotions in a safe and consensual environment. It is crucial to recognize that this type of roleplay may evoke real feelings of loss and grief, and thus should be approached with care.

Theoretical Framework

From a psychological standpoint, the exploration of grief through roleplay can be understood through several theories:

- **Attachment Theory:** This theory posits that individuals form emotional bonds that can influence their responses to loss. Roleplaying scenarios that involve pregnancy loss may allow participants to confront and process their attachment styles and the implications of loss in their relationships.

- **Grief Work:** The process of mourning often involves several stages, including denial, anger, bargaining, depression, and acceptance, as outlined by Kübler-Ross. Roleplaying can provide a structured way for individuals to navigate these stages, allowing for a deeper understanding of their emotional responses.

- **Catharsis:** Engaging in roleplay can serve as a cathartic experience, allowing individuals to express and release pent-up emotions associated with loss. This can facilitate healing and emotional growth.

Practical Considerations

When engaging in roleplay centered around pregnancy loss, it is essential to establish clear communication and consent. Here are some key points to consider:

1. **Pre-Roleplay Discussions:** Prior to engaging in any roleplay, partners should have open discussions about their feelings regarding pregnancy loss. This includes sharing personal experiences, discussing boundaries, and identifying any triggers that could lead to emotional distress.

2. **Setting Boundaries:** Clearly defined boundaries are crucial. Partners should discuss what aspects of pregnancy loss they are comfortable exploring and what topics or scenarios are off-limits. This may include specific language, actions, or emotional responses.

3. **Safewords and Check-Ins:** Establishing a safeword is vital for ensuring that both partners feel secure during the roleplay. Regular check-ins during the scenario can help gauge emotional responses and allow for adjustments as needed.

4. **Aftercare:** Aftercare is particularly important following a roleplay involving pregnancy loss. Partners should engage in comforting activities, such as cuddling, talking about the experience, or providing emotional support. This can help to process the emotions that arose during the roleplay and reinforce the bond between partners.

Examples of Roleplaying Scenarios

Here are some examples of scenarios that may be explored in the context of pregnancy loss roleplay:

- **The Miscarriage Scenario:** One partner may roleplay as someone who has just experienced a miscarriage, while the other partner provides support. This scenario can involve discussions about feelings of loss, guilt, and the impact on their relationship.

- **Stillbirth Roleplay:** In this scenario, partners may explore the emotional aftermath of stillbirth. This can include rituals of remembrance, discussing the impact on their lives, and navigating the complexities of grief together.

- **The Supportive Partner:** One partner may take on the role of a supportive figure, offering comfort and understanding to the grieving partner. This scenario can focus on the dynamics of support, empathy, and the challenges of navigating grief as a couple.

Addressing Potential Problems

While roleplaying pregnancy loss can be a powerful and cathartic experience, it is not without its challenges. Some potential problems include:

- **Emotional Overwhelm:** Participants may find themselves overwhelmed by emotions that arise during the roleplay. It is essential to have strategies in place for grounding oneself and returning to a state of emotional equilibrium.

- **Miscommunication:** Misunderstandings can occur if partners do not clearly communicate their feelings and boundaries. Regular discussions and check-ins can help mitigate this risk.

- **Triggering Past Trauma:** For individuals who have experienced pregnancy loss in real life, roleplaying these scenarios may trigger painful memories. It is crucial for partners to be aware of each other's histories and to approach the roleplay with sensitivity.

Conclusion

Roleplaying pregnancy loss and grief can be a profound means of exploring complex emotions and deepening intimacy between partners. By approaching the subject with care, establishing clear communication, and prioritizing aftercare, partners can create a safe space for emotional exploration. As with all aspects of breeding fantasy, the key lies in mutual consent, respect, and understanding.

Engaging in this type of roleplay not only allows for the exploration of grief but also fosters a deeper connection and understanding of each other's emotional landscapes. It is a testament to the power of intimacy and vulnerability in the realm of erotic roleplay.

Seeking support and therapy

In the realm of breeding fantasy and erotic pregnancy play, the emotional landscape can be complex and multifaceted. Engaging in such fantasies may evoke a range of feelings, from excitement and arousal to anxiety and guilt. Therefore, seeking support and therapy can be an essential step for individuals exploring these themes, particularly when navigating the psychological challenges that may arise.

Understanding the Need for Support

The first step in seeking support is recognizing the need for it. Individuals may experience emotional turbulence as they explore breeding fantasies, which can stem from societal taboos, personal insecurities, or past experiences. It is crucial to understand that these feelings are valid and that seeking help is a sign of strength rather than weakness.

Therapeutic Approaches

Several therapeutic approaches can be beneficial for individuals engaging with breeding fantasies:

- **Cognitive Behavioral Therapy (CBT):** CBT focuses on identifying and challenging negative thought patterns and behaviors. For those grappling with guilt or anxiety related to their fantasies, CBT can provide tools to reframe these thoughts and develop healthier coping strategies.

- **Sex Therapy:** A specialized branch of therapy that addresses sexual concerns, sex therapy can help individuals and couples discuss their fantasies openly and without judgment. This form of therapy can facilitate communication about desires, boundaries, and consent.

- **Support Groups:** Connecting with others who share similar interests can be incredibly validating. Support groups provide a safe space to discuss feelings, experiences, and challenges, fostering a sense of community and understanding.

- **Psychodynamic Therapy:** This approach delves into the unconscious motivations behind behaviors and fantasies. Understanding the roots of one's breeding fantasies can illuminate underlying issues, helping individuals to process complex emotions.

Identifying the Right Therapist

Finding a therapist who is knowledgeable and accepting of sexual diversity is crucial. Consider the following when searching for a therapist:

- **Experience with Kink and Fetish:** Look for therapists who have experience working with clients involved in kink and fetish communities. They should understand the nuances of these lifestyles and the importance of consent and boundaries.

- **Non-Judgmental Attitude:** A therapist should create a safe space for clients to express their fantasies without fear of judgment. This atmosphere of acceptance is vital for effective therapy.

- **Professional Credentials:** Ensure that the therapist is licensed and has appropriate credentials. It is also beneficial to check for any additional certifications in sex therapy or related fields.

Common Issues Addressed in Therapy

Individuals seeking therapy related to breeding fantasies may encounter various issues, including:

- **Guilt and Shame:** Many individuals feel guilt or shame regarding their fantasies, particularly if they conflict with societal norms. Therapy can help address these feelings and promote self-acceptance.

- **Anxiety and Fear:** Concerns about how others perceive their interests or fears about the implications of their fantasies can lead to anxiety. A therapist can assist in developing coping mechanisms to manage these fears.

- **Relationship Dynamics:** Breeding fantasies can impact intimate relationships, particularly if one partner is not on board. Therapy can facilitate open communication and help couples navigate these dynamics.

- **Trauma Processing:** For some, breeding fantasies may be intertwined with past traumas. Therapy provides a space to process these experiences and explore their impact on current fantasies and relationships.

Examples of Therapeutic Conversations

Here are a few hypothetical scenarios illustrating how therapy might unfold for individuals exploring breeding fantasies:

- **Scenario 1:** A client expresses guilt about their breeding fantasy, feeling it contradicts their desire for independence. The therapist guides the client in exploring the roots of this guilt, helping them to differentiate between societal expectations and personal desires.

- **Scenario 2:** A couple seeks therapy to address differing levels of interest in breeding play. Through guided conversations, they learn to articulate their desires and fears, ultimately finding common ground and establishing boundaries that honor both partners' comfort levels.

- **Scenario 3:** An individual discusses anxiety related to societal judgment of their fantasies. The therapist helps them develop strategies to cope with these feelings, including mindfulness techniques and role-playing scenarios to practice responses to potential judgment.

The Importance of Self-Care

In addition to therapy, incorporating self-care practices can enhance emotional well-being when exploring breeding fantasies. Consider the following self-care strategies:

- **Journaling:** Writing about feelings, fantasies, and experiences can provide clarity and insight, helping individuals process their emotions.

- **Mindfulness and Meditation:** Engaging in mindfulness practices can reduce anxiety and promote self-acceptance, allowing individuals to embrace their fantasies without fear.

- **Creative Expression:** Exploring breeding fantasies through art, writing, or other creative outlets can be therapeutic and fulfilling.

Conclusion

Seeking support and therapy is a vital aspect of navigating the complexities of breeding fantasy and erotic pregnancy play. By understanding the need for support, identifying the right therapeutic approaches, and addressing common issues, individuals can foster a healthier relationship with their fantasies.

Ultimately, therapy can facilitate personal growth, self-acceptance, and deeper intimacy in relationships, allowing individuals to explore their desires in a safe and supportive environment.

Balancing fantasy and reality

In the exploration of breeding fantasies, the line between erotic roleplay and reality can often become blurred. This section delves into the complexities of maintaining a healthy balance between the two, ensuring that participants can enjoy their fantasies without compromising their emotional well-being or real-life relationships.

The Importance of Balance

The concept of balance in erotic roleplay is essential for several reasons:

- **Emotional Well-being:** Engaging in breeding fantasies can evoke a wide range of emotions, from excitement and desire to anxiety and fear. Acknowledging these feelings and understanding their sources is crucial for maintaining mental health.
- **Relationship Dynamics:** When fantasies begin to influence real-life relationships, it is vital to communicate openly with partners. Misunderstandings can lead to feelings of jealousy, insecurity, or inadequacy if one partner feels pressured to fulfill a fantasy.
- **Psychological Safety:** Fantasy can serve as a safe space for exploring desires that may not align with one's everyday reality. However, it is essential to recognize when these fantasies might start to impact one's self-image or societal roles negatively.

Theoretical Frameworks

Several psychological theories can help in understanding the dynamics of balancing fantasy and reality:

Cognitive Dissonance Theory Cognitive dissonance theory posits that individuals experience discomfort when holding conflicting beliefs or engaging in behaviors that contradict their self-image. In the context of breeding fantasies, a participant may enjoy the thrill of the fantasy but feel guilt or shame afterward. This dissonance can lead to anxiety and affect the individual's overall mental health. To mitigate this, individuals can:

- Engage in self-reflection to understand the roots of their fantasies.
- Communicate openly with partners to align desires and expectations.
- Reframe their understanding of the fantasy as a legitimate expression of their sexuality.

Maslow's Hierarchy of Needs Maslow's hierarchy of needs suggests that individuals are motivated by a series of hierarchical needs, culminating in self-actualization. For those engaging in breeding fantasies, achieving a balance between fantasy and reality may involve addressing various needs:

- **Physiological Needs:** Ensure that basic physical needs are met before engaging in fantasy play.
- **Safety Needs:** Establish a safe and consensual environment for roleplay, including emotional safety.
- **Belongingness and Love Needs:** Foster connections with partners who understand and accept these fantasies, promoting healthy relationships.
- **Esteem Needs:** Engage in self-affirmation practices to counter feelings of guilt or shame associated with the fantasy.
- **Self-Actualization:** Encourage personal growth through exploration of fantasies in a way that aligns with one's values and beliefs.

Practical Strategies for Balancing Fantasy and Reality

To navigate the delicate balance between fantasy and reality, individuals can employ several practical strategies:

Open Communication Establishing a dialogue with partners about desires, boundaries, and feelings is crucial. This can include:

- Regular check-ins to discuss how each partner feels about their roleplay experiences.
- Sharing insights about what aspects of the fantasy are most enjoyable and which may cause discomfort.

Setting Clear Boundaries   Defining what is acceptable within the context of the fantasy can help prevent feelings of discomfort or coercion. This includes:

- Establishing clear safewords and signals to pause or stop the roleplay if it becomes overwhelming.
- Outlining specific scenarios that are off-limits to ensure that both partners feel safe and respected.

Incorporating Reality Checks   Integrating moments of reality into the fantasy can help ground participants and maintain a sense of perspective. This may involve:

- Taking breaks during roleplay to discuss feelings and reaffirm consent.
- Reminding each other of the distinction between fantasy and real-life responsibilities, especially if the roleplay begins to feel too intense.

Self-Reflection and Journaling   Encouraging self-reflection through journaling can help individuals process their thoughts and feelings about their fantasies. Questions to consider may include:

- What aspects of the fantasy resonate with my real-life desires?
- Are there any feelings of guilt or shame that I need to address?
- How can I communicate my needs and boundaries more effectively with my partner?

Examples of Balance in Practice

Consider a couple, Alex and Jamie, who engage in breeding fantasies. They have established a safe word and regularly check in with each other about their feelings. One evening, during a particularly intense roleplay session, Jamie begins to feel overwhelmed. They use their safeword, and the roleplay pauses. They take time to discuss what triggered Jamie's feelings and adjust their boundaries for future sessions. This open communication allows them to enjoy their fantasy while respecting each other's emotional limits.

In another scenario, a person may find themselves fantasizing about pregnancy in their everyday life, leading to feelings of anxiety about their current relationship status. They decide to seek therapy, where they explore the roots of their fantasy and how it relates to their self-image and societal expectations. Through this process, they learn to embrace their desires while developing a healthier relationship with their reality.

Conclusion

Balancing fantasy and reality in breeding play is a nuanced endeavor that requires self-awareness, communication, and ongoing negotiation. By understanding the psychological implications of their desires and employing practical strategies, individuals can create a fulfilling and healthy exploration of their breeding fantasies. Ultimately, the goal is to enjoy the thrill of fantasy while ensuring that it enhances rather than detracts from their overall well-being and relationships.

Addressing guilt and shame

Guilt and shame are powerful emotions that can significantly impact individuals engaging in breeding fantasy and erotic pregnancy play. Understanding these feelings, their origins, and how to address them is crucial for maintaining a healthy and consensual exploration of one's desires.

Understanding Guilt and Shame

Guilt is often experienced when one believes they have violated their own moral standards or the expectations of society. It can manifest as a feeling of remorse or responsibility for actions taken or not taken. In the context of breeding fantasy, guilt may arise from societal norms that stigmatize sexual desires, particularly those surrounding pregnancy and reproduction.

Shame, on the other hand, is a more profound emotional experience that relates to one's sense of self-worth. It is the feeling that one is fundamentally flawed or unworthy due to their desires or actions. Shame can be particularly potent in breeding fantasies, as it often intersects with deeply ingrained societal beliefs about sexuality, motherhood, and femininity.

Theoretical Perspectives

From a psychological standpoint, Brene Brown's research on vulnerability and shame provides valuable insights. Brown posits that shame thrives in secrecy and silence; it is often exacerbated by a lack of communication and understanding. Thus, addressing guilt and shame in breeding fantasy requires open dialogue and a supportive environment.

Furthermore, the theory of cognitive dissonance suggests that when individuals hold conflicting beliefs—such as enjoying a fantasy that society deems taboo—they may experience discomfort. This discomfort can lead to feelings of guilt and shame, prompting individuals to either suppress their desires or rationalize them in ways that align with societal norms.

Common Problems Associated with Guilt and Shame

1. **Internalized Stigma**: Many individuals internalize societal stigma surrounding non-normative sexual desires, leading to guilt over their fantasies. This internal conflict can hinder their ability to engage fully in the experience.

2. **Fear of Judgment**: The fear of being judged by peers or loved ones can amplify feelings of shame, making individuals hesitant to share their fantasies or seek support.

3. **Relationship Strain**: Guilt and shame can create barriers in communication between partners, leading to misunderstandings and emotional distance.

4. **Withdrawal from Community**: Individuals may isolate themselves from supportive communities due to feelings of shame, missing out on valuable resources and connections.

Strategies for Addressing Guilt and Shame

1. **Open Communication**: Encouraging honest discussions about desires, boundaries, and feelings can help alleviate guilt and shame. Partners should create a safe space for sharing without fear of judgment.

2. **Education and Understanding**: Learning about the psychological aspects of breeding fantasy can normalize these desires. Understanding that many people share similar fantasies can help mitigate feelings of isolation.

3. **Reframing Perspectives**: Individuals can work on reframing their thoughts surrounding their fantasies. Instead of viewing them as shameful, they can be seen as a natural part of human sexuality.

4. **Therapeutic Support**: Seeking therapy or counseling can provide a space to explore these feelings in depth. A therapist can help individuals process their emotions and develop coping strategies.

5. **Community Engagement**: Joining supportive communities, either online or in-person, can help individuals feel less alone. Sharing experiences with others who understand can reduce feelings of guilt and shame.

6. **Mindfulness and Self-Compassion**: Practicing mindfulness can help individuals observe their thoughts and feelings without judgment. Self-compassion techniques can foster a kinder internal dialogue, reducing the impact of guilt and shame.

Examples of Addressing Guilt and Shame

Consider a couple, Alex and Jamie, who are exploring breeding fantasies. Initially, Alex feels guilty about their desire to roleplay pregnancy, believing it contradicts their values. Through open communication, Jamie reassures Alex that their feelings are valid and that they can explore these fantasies together in a safe, consensual manner.

Over time, Alex learns about the psychological aspects of their desires and begins to reframe their thoughts. They join an online community where they connect with others who share similar interests, reducing their feelings of isolation. With the support of their partner and community, Alex develops a healthier relationship with their fantasies, leading to a more fulfilling exploration of their desires.

Conclusion

Addressing guilt and shame in breeding fantasy is an essential aspect of creating a healthy and enjoyable experience. By fostering open communication, understanding, and support, individuals can navigate these complex emotions and embrace their desires without fear. Ultimately, acknowledging and addressing guilt and shame can lead to deeper intimacy and connection with oneself and one's partner.

Exploring the role of power dynamics in mental health

Power dynamics play a crucial role in shaping our mental health, particularly within the context of erotic roleplay and breeding fantasies. Understanding these dynamics can illuminate how individuals navigate their desires, boundaries, and emotional landscapes. This section delves into the interplay between power, consent, and mental well-being, exploring both the positive and negative implications of power dynamics in the realm of breeding fantasy.

Theoretical Framework

The concept of power dynamics can be understood through various psychological and sociological lenses. One prominent theory is the *Power-Dependence Theory*, which posits that the power one holds in a relationship is contingent upon the dependence of the other party on that power. In the context of breeding fantasy, this dependence may manifest in the desire for intimacy, validation, or emotional support.

Furthermore, *Foucault's theory of power* suggests that power is not merely repressive but can also be productive. In erotic roleplay, power dynamics can create spaces for individuals to explore their identities and desires in ways that may not be possible in their everyday lives. This exploration can foster a sense of agency, allowing participants to reclaim narratives around sexuality, reproduction, and intimacy.

Positive Aspects of Power Dynamics

In the context of breeding fantasies, power dynamics can facilitate deeper connections and enhance emotional intimacy. Engaging in consensual power exchange can lead to the following positive outcomes:

- **Enhanced Communication:** Clear communication about desires, boundaries, and fantasies can lead to a stronger bond between partners. When individuals feel empowered to express their needs, it fosters an environment of trust and safety.

- **Exploration of Identity:** Power dynamics allow individuals to explore different facets of their identity. For example, one partner may take on a dominant role, allowing them to embrace assertiveness, while the other partner may explore submission, leading to self-discovery and personal growth.

- **Emotional Release:** Engaging in power dynamics can provide an emotional outlet. Participants may experience catharsis through roleplay, allowing them to process complex feelings related to sexuality, reproduction, and societal expectations.

Challenges and Risks of Power Dynamics

Despite the potential benefits, power dynamics also carry inherent risks, particularly if not navigated with care. Some challenges include:

- **Miscommunication:** Power dynamics can lead to misunderstandings if boundaries are not clearly established. This miscommunication can result in feelings of violation or discomfort, undermining the trust necessary for healthy roleplay.

+ **Emotional Vulnerability:** Engaging in breeding fantasies can evoke deep-seated emotions related to fertility, parenthood, or societal pressures. If these emotions are not addressed, they may lead to anxiety, depression, or feelings of inadequacy.

+ **Reinforcement of Negative Patterns:** For some individuals, engaging in power dynamics may inadvertently reinforce negative mental health patterns. For example, a person with a history of trauma may find themselves re-enacting harmful dynamics, leading to further emotional distress.

Examples and Case Studies

To illustrate the role of power dynamics in mental health, consider the following hypothetical scenarios:

+ **Scenario 1:** A couple engages in breeding roleplay where one partner assumes a dominant role, expressing the desire to "impregnate" the other. This dynamic is consensual, and both partners have communicated their boundaries. The dominant partner feels empowered and validated, while the submissive partner experiences a sense of safety and trust. This scenario highlights the potential for positive emotional outcomes when power dynamics are navigated thoughtfully.

+ **Scenario 2:** In contrast, another couple may engage in similar roleplay, but one partner has not fully expressed their discomfort with certain aspects of the fantasy. The dominant partner, unaware of these feelings, pushes boundaries, leading to feelings of violation for the submissive partner. This scenario underscores the importance of ongoing communication and the potential risks of power dynamics when consent is not fully informed.

Strategies for Navigating Power Dynamics

To ensure that power dynamics contribute positively to mental health, individuals should consider the following strategies:

+ **Establish Clear Boundaries:** Before engaging in any roleplay, partners should discuss their limits and boundaries. This discussion should include potential emotional triggers and safe words to ensure that both parties feel secure.

- **Regular Check-Ins:** During and after roleplay, partners should engage in regular check-ins to assess each other's emotional state. This practice fosters open communication and allows for adjustments to be made as necessary.

- **Prioritize Aftercare:** Aftercare is essential in any power exchange dynamic. Providing emotional support and reassurance after roleplay can help partners process their experiences and reinforce feelings of safety and connection.

- **Seek Professional Support:** If individuals find themselves struggling with the emotional implications of power dynamics, seeking the guidance of a mental health professional can be beneficial. Therapy can provide a safe space for exploring feelings and developing coping strategies.

Conclusion

Exploring the role of power dynamics in mental health within the context of breeding fantasy reveals a complex interplay of consent, identity, and emotional well-being. While power dynamics can enhance intimacy and foster self-exploration, they also carry risks that must be navigated with care. By prioritizing communication, establishing boundaries, and engaging in aftercare, individuals can cultivate a healthy relationship with their fantasies, ultimately enriching their emotional and mental health.

Incorporating self-care into the fantasy

In the realm of breeding fantasy and erotic pregnancy play, self-care is an essential component that ensures both mental and emotional well-being. Engaging in such intimate and often taboo explorations can evoke a spectrum of feelings, from exhilaration to anxiety. Therefore, embedding self-care practices into these fantasies not only enhances the experience but also safeguards against potential emotional pitfalls.

Understanding Self-Care in Fantasy Contexts

Self-care refers to the intentional practices that individuals engage in to promote their own physical, mental, and emotional health. Within the context of breeding fantasy, self-care can be understood through various lenses:

- **Physical Self-Care:** This involves maintaining one's physical health, which is especially pertinent when engaging in roleplay scenarios that may mimic pregnancy or childbirth. It includes practices such as regular exercise, balanced nutrition, and adequate rest.

- **Emotional Self-Care:** Engaging in breeding fantasies can stir deep-seated emotions, including desires, fears, and societal judgments. Emotional self-care involves recognizing and processing these feelings through journaling, therapy, or open discussions with partners.

- **Mental Self-Care:** This entails stimulating the mind and fostering a positive mindset. Techniques such as mindfulness, meditation, and positive affirmations can help individuals maintain a healthy mental state while navigating complex fantasies.

Theoretical Perspectives on Self-Care

From a psychological standpoint, self-care is crucial for maintaining a healthy relationship with one's desires. According to the Self-Determination Theory (SDT), which posits that individuals are motivated by intrinsic and extrinsic factors, self-care practices can enhance intrinsic motivation by fostering a sense of autonomy and competence. This is particularly relevant in breeding fantasy, where individuals may grapple with feelings of vulnerability and dependence.

Practical Self-Care Strategies in Breeding Fantasy

Incorporating self-care into breeding fantasies can be achieved through various strategies:

1. **Pre-Roleplay Preparation:** Before engaging in roleplay, individuals should take time to ground themselves. This can include meditative practices or engaging in activities that bring joy and relaxation, such as taking a bath or enjoying a favorite hobby.

2. **Setting Boundaries:** Clearly defining boundaries before entering a fantasy scenario is vital. This includes discussing what aspects of the fantasy are comfortable and what may be triggering. Having a mutual understanding creates a safe space for exploration.

3. **Post-Roleplay Reflection:** After a roleplay session, individuals should engage in a debriefing process. This can involve discussing what was enjoyable, what felt uncomfortable, and how the experience aligns with their emotional state. This reflection can help in processing the experience and integrating it into their self-concept.

4. **Incorporating Aftercare:** Aftercare is an integral part of BDSM and kink practices that can be applied to breeding fantasy. It involves providing physical and emotional support to partners after roleplay, ensuring that both parties feel secure and cared for. This can include cuddling, verbal reassurance, or simply spending quiet time together.

5. **Creating a Self-Care Ritual:** Establishing a personal self-care ritual that aligns with the fantasy can enhance the experience. For instance, incorporating aromatherapy with scents associated with comfort and relaxation can create a soothing atmosphere that balances the intensity of the fantasy.

Addressing Challenges and Emotional Triggers

While engaging in breeding fantasy, individuals may encounter emotional triggers related to their own experiences with pregnancy, loss, or societal expectations. It is essential to recognize these triggers and have strategies in place to address them. For instance, if a partner feels overwhelmed during a roleplay scenario, they should feel empowered to use a safeword or pause the session for a check-in.

Furthermore, it is beneficial to have a plan for emotional support. This can include having a trusted friend or therapist to talk to about feelings that arise from the fantasies. Engaging in community forums or support groups can also provide a sense of belonging and understanding.

Conclusion

Incorporating self-care into breeding fantasy is not merely an afterthought; it is a fundamental aspect that enriches the experience and promotes overall well-being. By prioritizing self-care, individuals can navigate the complexities of their desires with confidence and security, ultimately leading to a more fulfilling exploration of their fantasies. Embracing self-care practices allows for a deeper connection to oneself and one's partner, fostering intimacy and trust in the journey of erotic exploration.

$$\text{Self-Care} = \text{Physical Care} + \text{Emotional Care} + \text{Mental Care} \quad (13)$$

As individuals engage in breeding fantasies, let this equation serve as a reminder that self-care is the foundation upon which enjoyable and fulfilling experiences are built.

Beyond the Bedroom: Integrating Breeding Fantasy into Daily Life

Communication and Consent

Maintaining open communication

Open communication is the cornerstone of any healthy relationship, particularly when exploring sensitive and potentially taboo topics such as breeding fantasy and erotic pregnancy play. This section will delve into the theoretical underpinnings of communication, the common challenges faced, and practical strategies to foster a communicative environment that prioritizes consent, understanding, and emotional safety.

Theoretical Framework

Communication theory suggests that effective communication encompasses several key components: clarity, active listening, empathy, and feedback. According to the *Transactional Model of Communication*, communication is a dynamic process where both parties engage in sending and receiving messages, often simultaneously. This model emphasizes that communication is not merely about exchanging words but involves interpreting and responding to nonverbal cues, emotional states, and contextual factors.

$$C = S + R + E \tag{14}$$

Where:

- C = Communication

- S = Sender's message

- R = Receiver's interpretation

- E = Environmental context

In the context of breeding fantasy, the emotional stakes are high, and misunderstandings can lead to feelings of discomfort or violation. Therefore, establishing a framework for open communication is crucial.

Common Challenges

Despite the importance of open communication, several challenges can arise:

- **Fear of Judgment:** Individuals may hesitate to express their fantasies due to fear of being judged or misunderstood by their partner. This fear can stem from societal stigmas surrounding breeding fantasies and pregnancy play.

- **Misinterpretation:** The nuances of language can lead to misinterpretation of intentions. For instance, a playful comment about pregnancy may be taken seriously, creating tension.

- **Power Dynamics:** In BDSM and kink relationships, power imbalances can complicate communication. A submissive partner may feel pressured to agree to scenarios they are uncomfortable with, fearing it may disappoint their dominant partner.

- **Emotional Triggers:** Discussions about pregnancy can evoke strong emotional responses, particularly for individuals who have experienced loss or trauma. This can make open communication difficult.

Strategies for Open Communication

To foster an environment of open communication, consider the following strategies:

- **Establish Safe Spaces:** Create a physical and emotional space where both partners feel safe to express their thoughts and feelings without fear of judgment. This might involve setting aside specific times to discuss fantasies or concerns.

- **Use "I" Statements:** Encourage the use of "I" statements to express feelings and desires. For example, saying "I feel excited when I think about trying to conceive" rather than "You should want to try to conceive" can reduce defensiveness and promote understanding.

- **Active Listening:** Practice active listening techniques, such as paraphrasing what your partner has said to ensure understanding. This not only clarifies the message but also shows that you value their perspective.

   "What I hear you saying is that you're excited about the idea of exploring this fantasy, but you're also concerned about how it might affect our relationship."

- **Regular Check-Ins:** Schedule regular check-ins to discuss feelings about the roleplay. This can be a dedicated time where both partners can express any concerns or desires that have arisen since the last discussion.

- **Educate Together:** Engage in educational activities together, such as reading literature on breeding fantasies or attending workshops. This can help normalize the conversation and provide a shared knowledge base.

- **Normalize Vulnerability:** Acknowledge that discussing fantasies can be vulnerable. Encourage openness by sharing your own feelings of vulnerability and inviting your partner to do the same.

Examples of Open Communication in Practice

To illustrate these strategies in action, consider the following scenarios:

- **Scenario 1: Expressing Excitement and Fear**

   Partner A expresses excitement about exploring a breeding fantasy but also shares a fear of potential pregnancy. They say, "I've been thinking about how thrilling it would be to roleplay trying to conceive, but I'm also scared about the reality of pregnancy. Can we talk about how we can make this fantasy enjoyable while addressing my concerns?"

   Partner B responds with empathy, "I understand that this is a big step for you. Let's discuss what boundaries we can set to ensure you feel comfortable while exploring this fantasy."

- Scenario 2: Addressing Misinterpretation

    During a roleplay session, Partner B playfully suggests a scenario that unintentionally triggers Partner A's anxiety about pregnancy loss. Recognizing the discomfort, Partner B pauses the roleplay and asks, "I noticed you seemed upset when I mentioned that. Can we talk about how that made you feel?"

    Partner A replies, "It reminded me of a difficult experience I had. I appreciate you checking in. Let's adjust the scenario to avoid that."

- Scenario 3: Regular Check-Ins

    After a few roleplay sessions, both partners agree to have a monthly check-in. During this meeting, they discuss what they enjoyed, any discomforts, and new fantasies they want to explore. Partner A says, "I loved our last roleplay, but I felt a bit overwhelmed by the intensity. Can we dial it back a little next time?"

    Partner B responds, "Absolutely, let's find a balance that works for both of us."

Conclusion

Maintaining open communication is essential for the healthy exploration of breeding fantasies. By understanding the theoretical foundations of communication, recognizing common challenges, and implementing effective strategies, partners can create a safe and consensual environment that fosters intimacy and trust. This commitment to communication not only enhances the roleplay experience but also strengthens the overall relationship, allowing both partners to explore their desires with confidence and security.

Consenting to public roleplaying and displays of pregnancy

Public roleplaying and displays of pregnancy can be thrilling experiences that extend the boundaries of intimacy and fantasy into the outside world. However, such practices must be approached with careful consideration of consent, boundaries, and the potential implications for all parties involved. This section will explore the nuances of consenting to public displays of pregnancy, addressing relevant theories, potential problems, and practical examples.

Theoretical Framework

The foundation of any public roleplay scenario lies in the principles of consent and communication. Consent is not merely a one-time agreement but a continuous dialogue that evolves as the context changes. According to [?], consent in intimate relationships must encompass not only the act itself but also the setting in which it occurs. This means that both partners must feel comfortable with the idea of engaging in public displays of pregnancy, understanding that such actions may elicit various responses from onlookers.

Moreover, [?] emphasizes the importance of context in erotic experiences. The thrill of public displays often stems from the risk associated with being observed. This risk can heighten arousal but must be balanced with the potential for discomfort or harm. Thus, establishing clear boundaries and guidelines for public roleplay is essential to ensure that both partners can enjoy the experience without feeling vulnerable or exposed in an undesirable way.

Problems and Considerations

While the allure of public roleplay is undeniable, there are several challenges that couples may face:

- **Public Perception:** Engaging in public displays of pregnancy can attract attention, and not all reactions will be positive. Couples must consider the societal norms and values of their environment. What may be acceptable in one community could be met with disdain or hostility in another.

- **Consent from Bystanders:** Public roleplay inevitably involves other people who have not consented to be part of the scenario. This raises ethical questions about their comfort and boundaries. It is essential to be mindful of the reactions of those around you and to avoid scenarios that may intrude on their personal space.

- **Safety Concerns:** Public displays can sometimes lead to unwanted attention or harassment. Couples should have a plan in place to address any uncomfortable situations that may arise. This could include identifying safe spaces to retreat to or having a predetermined signal to indicate discomfort.

- **Emotional Impact:** The emotional ramifications of public roleplay can vary widely. While some may find it exhilarating, others may experience anxiety or fear. It is crucial to have open discussions about these feelings before engaging in public displays.

Examples of Public Roleplaying Scenarios

To illustrate the concept of consenting to public roleplaying and displays of pregnancy, consider the following scenarios:

- **Costumed Events:** Participating in a themed event, such as a convention or festival, allows couples to engage in roleplay within a context that is generally more accepting of unique expressions of identity. For example, a couple may choose to dress in costumes that reflect their breeding fantasy, creating a playful and consensual atmosphere.

- **Private Gatherings:** Hosting or attending a private party where like-minded individuals are present can provide a safe space for public displays. Here, participants can negotiate the boundaries of their roleplay and ensure that everyone involved is comfortable with the scenario.

- **Public Parks or Beaches:** Some couples may enjoy the thrill of engaging in roleplay in more public settings, such as parks or beaches. It is vital to choose less crowded areas and to remain aware of the comfort levels of those nearby. Couples should discuss their boundaries beforehand and establish a signal to indicate if one partner feels uncomfortable.

- **Social Media and Online Platforms:** In the digital age, public roleplay can extend to online platforms where individuals can share their fantasies and experiences with a wider audience. Couples may choose to create content that reflects their breeding fantasies, ensuring that all parties involved have consented to the sharing of personal information and images.

Conclusion

Consenting to public roleplaying and displays of pregnancy is an intricate dance that requires clear communication, mutual respect, and a deep understanding of the emotional and social implications involved. By prioritizing consent, establishing boundaries, and remaining mindful of the reactions of others, couples can explore the exhilarating world of public displays while maintaining a safe and supportive environment for their fantasies. As with any aspect of erotic play, the key lies in open dialogue and a shared commitment to ensuring that both partners feel empowered and respected in their choices.

Discussing Boundaries with Others

In the realm of breeding fantasy and erotic pregnancy play, discussing boundaries with others is not merely a formality; it is a crucial step that ensures the safety, comfort, and satisfaction of all participants involved. This discourse can be complex, laden with the nuances of personal feelings, societal norms, and the inherent nature of the fantasies themselves.

Understanding Boundaries

Boundaries can be defined as the limits we set for ourselves and others in terms of behavior, emotions, and physical interactions. In the context of erotic roleplay, boundaries may encompass what is acceptable in terms of language, physical touch, and the extent to which one wishes to engage in certain scenarios. The concept of boundaries is essential for maintaining a healthy dynamic, particularly in scenarios that involve power exchange, such as dominance and submission.

The Importance of Clear Communication

Effective communication is the cornerstone of any healthy relationship, especially when it comes to discussing boundaries. Clear communication fosters an environment where participants feel safe to express their desires and limitations without fear of judgment or coercion. This can be achieved through open dialogue, where each party is encouraged to share their thoughts and feelings regarding their fantasies and the boundaries they wish to establish.

Techniques for Discussing Boundaries

1. **Active Listening**: When discussing boundaries, it is vital to practice active listening. This means fully concentrating on what the other person is saying, understanding their message, and responding thoughtfully. This technique helps to validate feelings and encourages a more profound connection.

2. **Use of 'I' Statements**: Framing thoughts in terms of personal feelings can prevent the other party from feeling attacked or defensive. For example, saying "I feel uncomfortable when..." rather than "You make me uncomfortable when..." can facilitate a more constructive conversation.

3. **Roleplay Scenarios**: Engaging in roleplay scenarios that are less intense can serve as a practice ground for discussing boundaries. For instance, participants might roleplay a scenario where they are discussing their everyday limits, which can transition into more intimate discussions about their breeding fantasies.

4. **Written Agreements**: For some, putting boundaries in writing can provide clarity and serve as a reference point. This can include a list of do's and don'ts, which can be revisited and revised as necessary.

Common Problems in Boundary Discussions

While discussing boundaries is essential, it can also present challenges. Here are some common issues that may arise:

1. **Fear of Rejection**: Participants may worry that expressing their boundaries will lead to rejection or disappointment from their partner. This fear can stifle open communication and lead to misunderstandings.

2. **Misinterpretation**: Boundaries can sometimes be misinterpreted, leading to unintentional violations. It is crucial for all parties to ensure they have a mutual understanding of what has been discussed.

3. **Power Imbalances**: In dynamics involving dominance and submission, power imbalances can complicate boundary discussions. The submissive partner may feel pressured to agree to boundaries that they are uncomfortable with due to their desire to please the dominant partner.

4. **Cultural and Societal Influences**: Societal norms and cultural backgrounds can influence how individuals perceive boundaries. It is vital to recognize these influences and approach discussions with sensitivity and respect for differing viewpoints.

Examples of Boundary Discussions

To illustrate the process of discussing boundaries, consider the following hypothetical scenarios:

- **Scenario 1**: Alex and Jamie are exploring breeding fantasies. Alex expresses a desire to roleplay a scenario involving natural conception. Jamie is unsure and feels uncomfortable with the idea of portraying pregnancy. They sit down together and have an open discussion about their feelings, ultimately agreeing to explore the fantasy in a way that feels safe for both, perhaps by incorporating elements of fantasy without actual physical implications.

- **Scenario 2**: Taylor and Morgan have been engaging in breeding roleplay, but Taylor begins to feel overwhelmed by the intensity of the scenarios. They decide to have a conversation where Taylor uses 'I' statements to express their feelings. Morgan listens actively and reassures Taylor that their comfort is the priority, leading to a renegotiation of their roleplay limits.

Conclusion

Discussing boundaries with others in the context of breeding fantasy and erotic pregnancy play is an essential practice that fosters trust, safety, and mutual satisfaction. By employing effective communication techniques and being aware of the potential challenges, participants can navigate these discussions with greater ease. Ultimately, the goal is to create a shared understanding that respects individual limits while allowing for the exploration of desires within a safe and consensual framework.

In this way, the act of discussing boundaries becomes not just a necessary task but a vital part of the erotic journey, enhancing intimacy and connection between partners while paving the way for more fulfilling and pleasurable experiences.

Educating friends and family members

In the realm of breeding fantasy and erotic pregnancy play, open communication extends beyond the bedroom and into our social circles. Educating friends and family members about these interests can foster understanding, reduce stigma, and create a supportive environment for individuals who engage in such fantasies. This process, however, is not without its challenges. It requires sensitivity, awareness of social dynamics, and a commitment to respectful dialogue.

Understanding the Need for Education

The first step in educating friends and family is recognizing why this education is necessary. Many people harbor misconceptions about fetishes and kinks, often viewing them through the lens of societal taboos. Breeding fantasy, in particular, can elicit strong reactions due to its associations with fertility, motherhood, and sexuality. By educating those around us, we can help dismantle these misconceptions and promote a more nuanced understanding of our desires.

Theoretical Frameworks

To effectively educate friends and family, it is beneficial to employ certain theoretical frameworks. The **Social Learning Theory** posits that behaviors are learned through observation and imitation. By sharing our experiences and explaining the motivations behind our interests, we can help others understand that these fantasies do not define our entire identities but are rather a part of our complex human sexuality.

Additionally, **Intersectionality** can be a useful lens through which to view our discussions. This framework acknowledges that individuals experience overlapping social identities, such as race, gender, and sexuality, which can affect their perspectives on breeding fantasies. Recognizing these intersections can help tailor our conversations to resonate with our audience's unique experiences and beliefs.

Strategies for Educating Others

1. **Choose the Right Time and Place:** Timing is crucial when discussing sensitive topics. Opt for a private and comfortable setting where everyone feels safe to express their thoughts and feelings. Avoid initiating these conversations during tense or inappropriate moments.

2. **Use Clear and Respectful Language:** When discussing breeding fantasies, use language that is clear and respectful. Avoid jargon that may alienate or confuse your audience. Instead, focus on explaining the fantasy in a relatable manner, emphasizing that it is a consensual and safe exploration of desires.

3. **Share Personal Experiences:** Personal anecdotes can be powerful tools for education. By sharing your journey into breeding fantasy, you can humanize the experience and make it more relatable. Discuss how this fantasy enhances intimacy and connection in your relationships, reinforcing that it is not merely about sexual gratification.

4. **Address Misconceptions:** Be prepared to confront common misconceptions. Many people may assume that breeding fantasies are inherently linked to a desire for actual pregnancy or that they reflect a lack of maturity. Clarify that these fantasies can exist independently of real-life desires and that they often stem from a complex interplay of psychological factors.

5. **Encourage Questions:** Foster an open dialogue by encouraging friends and family to ask questions. This not only demonstrates your willingness to engage in the conversation but also provides an opportunity to clarify misunderstandings and dispel myths.

6. **Provide Resources:** Offer educational resources, such as articles, books, or documentaries, that delve into the psychology of fetishes and the nuances of breeding fantasy. This can help your audience gain a broader understanding and context for your interests.

Handling Reactions

It is essential to prepare for a range of reactions when discussing breeding fantasy. Some individuals may respond with curiosity and support, while others may express discomfort or even disapproval. Here are some strategies for navigating these reactions:

- **Stay Calm and Composed:** If faced with negative reactions, maintain your composure. Responding with anger or defensiveness can escalate the situation. Instead, calmly reiterate your points and express your hope for understanding.

- **Acknowledge Their Feelings:** Recognize that your friends and family may have their own feelings and biases about breeding fantasies. Acknowledging their discomfort can create a more empathetic dialogue and encourage them to express their thoughts without fear of judgment.

- **Set Boundaries:** If a conversation becomes overly hostile or uncomfortable, it is perfectly acceptable to set boundaries. Politely indicate that you value their opinion but that certain topics may be off-limits for discussion.

Examples of Successful Conversations

To illustrate the effectiveness of these strategies, consider the following examples:

- **Example 1:** Sarah, a 30-year-old woman, decided to share her interest in breeding fantasy with her close friends during a casual dinner. She chose a relaxed environment and began by discussing the emotional aspects of her fantasy, highlighting how it enhances her relationship with her partner. Her friends responded positively, asking questions that led to a deeper understanding of her desires.

- **Example 2:** John, a 28-year-old man, faced skepticism from his family when he mentioned his interest in breeding fantasy. He prepared by gathering resources and discussing the psychological aspects of fetishes. Although his family was initially uncomfortable, they appreciated his effort to educate them and eventually became more accepting of his interests.

Conclusion

Educating friends and family members about breeding fantasy is a vital step in fostering understanding and acceptance. By employing clear communication, theoretical frameworks, and effective strategies, individuals can create a supportive environment that embraces diverse sexual interests. While challenges may arise, the potential for deeper connections and reduced stigma makes the effort worthwhile. Ultimately, open dialogue can lead to a greater appreciation of the complexities of human sexuality and the myriad ways individuals choose to express their desires.

Handling public judgment and stigma

Engaging in breeding fantasies and erotic pregnancy play can evoke a range of responses from those around us. While the intimate world of such fantasies can be a source of pleasure and connection between consenting partners, the reality of public judgment and societal stigma can create significant challenges for individuals who wish to explore these desires openly. This section aims to provide insight into the nature of public judgment, the stigma associated with breeding fantasies, and strategies for navigating these complexities.

Understanding Public Judgment

Public judgment often stems from societal norms and cultural beliefs that dictate acceptable behaviors and fantasies. Breeding fantasies may be perceived as taboo due to their association with procreation, sexuality, and the complexities of gender roles. The fear of being judged can lead individuals to conceal their interests, resulting in feelings of shame and isolation.

The Nature of Stigma

Stigma can manifest in various forms, including social, internalized, and institutional stigma. Social stigma refers to the negative perceptions held by society regarding certain behaviors or identities. Internalized stigma occurs when individuals adopt these negative beliefs about themselves, leading to feelings of unworthiness or shame. Institutional stigma can arise from policies or practices that discriminate against individuals based on their sexual preferences or identities.

Theoretical Frameworks

Several theoretical frameworks can help us understand the dynamics of public judgment and stigma in the context of breeding fantasies:

- **Labeling Theory:** This sociological perspective posits that individuals may be labeled based on their behaviors, leading to a self-fulfilling prophecy where they internalize these labels and act accordingly. For example, a person who enjoys breeding fantasies may be labeled as deviant, which can affect their self-image and relationships.

- **Social Identity Theory:** This theory suggests that individuals derive part of their self-concept from their membership in social groups. Those who engage in breeding fantasies may find themselves at odds with mainstream societal values, leading to a diminished sense of belonging and increased stigma.

- Intersectionality: This framework highlights how various social identities (e.g., gender, sexuality, race) intersect to create unique experiences of oppression or privilege. For example, a woman who expresses her breeding fantasies may face different societal judgments than a man who does the same, shaped by cultural expectations around femininity and masculinity.

Common Problems Associated with Public Judgment

Individuals who engage in breeding fantasies may encounter several problems related to public judgment, including:

- Fear of Exposure: The fear of being discovered can lead to anxiety and stress, causing individuals to hide their interests even from close friends or partners. This can hinder open communication and intimacy.

- Isolation: Stigmatization can result in social isolation, as individuals may withdraw from social interactions to avoid judgment. This can exacerbate feelings of loneliness and shame.

- Impact on Relationships: Public judgment can strain relationships, particularly if one partner is more open about their fantasies than the other. Discrepancies in comfort levels regarding public expression can lead to misunderstandings and conflicts.

Strategies for Navigating Public Judgment and Stigma

To effectively manage public judgment and stigma, individuals can adopt several strategies:

- Educate and Advocate: Increasing awareness about breeding fantasies and the importance of consent can help challenge societal norms. Engaging in discussions or sharing resources can foster understanding and reduce stigma.

- Find Supportive Communities: Connecting with like-minded individuals through online forums, local meetups, or workshops can provide a sense of belonging and validation. Support groups can offer a safe space to share experiences and strategies for coping with stigma.

- **Practice Self-Compassion:** Recognizing that desires and fantasies are a natural part of human sexuality can help individuals cultivate self-acceptance. Practicing self-compassion can mitigate the effects of internalized stigma and enhance emotional resilience.

- **Set Boundaries:** Establishing clear boundaries with friends and family regarding discussions about personal fantasies can protect individuals from unwanted judgment. It is essential to communicate comfort levels and respect each other's privacy.

- **Role-Play Scenarios in Safe Spaces:** Engaging in breeding fantasies within safe, consensual environments allows individuals to explore their desires without fear of judgment. This can enhance intimacy and reduce anxiety associated with public exposure.

- **Utilize Humor and Light-heartedness:** Approaching discussions about breeding fantasies with humor can diffuse tension and make the topic more approachable. This can help mitigate serious judgments and foster open conversations.

Conclusion

Handling public judgment and stigma surrounding breeding fantasies requires a multifaceted approach that emphasizes education, community support, and self-acceptance. By understanding the dynamics of stigma and employing strategies to navigate public perceptions, individuals can create a more fulfilling and authentic experience in their exploration of erotic pregnancy play. Embracing one's desires in a safe and consensual manner ultimately fosters deeper connections and enhances the overall experience of intimacy and pleasure.

The ethics of public roleplay

Public roleplay, particularly in the context of breeding fantasies, presents a unique set of ethical considerations that require careful navigation. Engaging in such activities outside the privacy of one's home can elicit a spectrum of reactions from the public, ranging from intrigue to discomfort, and even hostility. This section will explore the ethical dimensions of public roleplay, focusing on consent, societal norms, and the potential impact on both participants and bystanders.

Consent and Awareness

The cornerstone of any ethical roleplay is consent, which becomes even more complex in public settings. The principle of informed consent extends beyond the participants to include bystanders who may inadvertently become part of the scene. It is crucial to recognize that not everyone in a public space is consenting to witness or be involved in a roleplay scenario.

$$\text{Informed Consent} = \text{Awareness} + \text{Voluntariness} + \text{Competence} \quad (15)$$

Here, *Awareness* refers to the understanding of the roleplay context, *Voluntariness* indicates that participation or observation is not coerced, and *Competence* signifies that all parties involved are capable of giving consent.

To ethically engage in public roleplay, participants must consider the following:

- **Setting Boundaries:** Define clear boundaries about what is acceptable in public spaces. This includes discussing how far the roleplay can go without infringing on the comfort of others.

- **Choosing Appropriate Venues:** Select locations that are more accepting of alternative lifestyles, such as fetish events or LGBTQ+ friendly spaces, where the likelihood of encountering understanding audiences is higher.

- **Observing Reactions:** Be attentive to the reactions of bystanders. If discomfort is evident, it may be necessary to pause or alter the roleplay to respect their boundaries.

Societal Norms and Public Perception

Engaging in breeding fantasy roleplay in public can challenge societal norms and provoke strong reactions. The societal perception of pregnancy and breeding often carries significant weight, as they are tied to deeply ingrained cultural narratives about family, sexuality, and morality.

$$\text{Public Reaction} = f(\text{Cultural Norms}, \text{Context}, \text{Visibility}) \quad (16)$$

In this equation, *Cultural Norms* represent the prevailing attitudes towards sexuality and public displays of affection, *Context* refers to the specific setting in which the roleplay occurs, and *Visibility* indicates how apparent the roleplay is to passersby.

For example, a roleplay scenario involving pregnancy in a family-friendly park may provoke outrage, while the same scenario at a fetish convention may be celebrated. Understanding the nuances of context and visibility is essential for ethical public roleplay.

Impact on Bystanders

The ethical implications of public roleplay extend to the impact on bystanders. It is important to consider how the roleplay may affect those who are not participants.

- **Potential Distress:** Some individuals may feel uncomfortable or distressed witnessing public displays of sexual or fetishistic behavior. This discomfort can stem from personal beliefs, past experiences, or cultural conditioning.

- **Normalizing Fetishes:** On the other hand, public roleplay can also serve to normalize alternative sexual expressions. When done respectfully, it can educate bystanders about the diversity of human sexuality and foster a more accepting environment.

- **Creating Dialogue:** Ethical public roleplay can open avenues for conversation about sexuality, consent, and personal freedom. Engaging with bystanders who express curiosity can transform potentially negative encounters into opportunities for education.

Navigating Ethical Dilemmas

Participants in public roleplay may encounter ethical dilemmas that require thoughtful consideration. For instance, if a bystander approaches and expresses discomfort, participants must decide whether to continue or halt their roleplay.

In such cases, it is essential to weigh the right to express one's sexuality against the responsibility to respect the feelings of others. A practical approach might involve:

- **Immediate Check-ins:** If someone appears uncomfortable, participants should check in with each other and the bystander to assess the situation.

- **Flexibility:** Be willing to adapt the roleplay or relocate to a more suitable environment if necessary.

- **Exit Strategies:** Have a plan for gracefully exiting the situation if it becomes untenable for any party involved.

Conclusion

The ethics of public roleplay, particularly concerning breeding fantasies, necessitates a nuanced understanding of consent, societal norms, and the impact on bystanders. By prioritizing informed consent, being aware of cultural contexts, and respecting the feelings of others, participants can engage in public roleplay in a manner that is both fulfilling and ethically sound. Ultimately, the goal should be to create a space where all individuals can express their desires without infringing on the rights and comfort of others, fostering an atmosphere of mutual respect and understanding.

Fantasy Enhancement Techniques

Erotic storytelling and role-playing scenarios

Erotic storytelling and role-playing scenarios serve as powerful tools for individuals and couples exploring breeding fantasies. These practices not only enhance intimacy but also allow for the creation of rich narratives that can bring fantasies to life in a safe and consensual manner. This section delves into the significance of erotic storytelling, the construction of role-playing scenarios, and the psychological and emotional benefits they provide.

The Power of Narrative

Narratives have been used throughout human history to convey experiences, desires, and fantasies. In the context of eroticism, storytelling becomes a vehicle through which individuals can express their deepest desires and explore their fantasies without the constraints of reality. According to [?], storytelling in intimacy fosters a sense of connection and vulnerability, allowing partners to share their fantasies openly.

$$E = mc^2 \tag{17}$$

This equation, while primarily associated with physics, can metaphorically represent the energy exchange in erotic storytelling: the energy (E) of the narrative is influenced by the mass (m) of the emotions and desires involved, and the speed of light (c) symbolizes the intensity of the connection between partners.

Constructing Role-Playing Scenarios

Creating effective role-playing scenarios requires careful thought and consideration. Here are some steps to guide the process:

1. **Identify Fantasies:** Begin by discussing personal fantasies related to breeding. This could include scenarios involving natural conception, artificial insemination, or even postpartum dynamics.

2. **Set the Scene:** Choose a setting that enhances the fantasy. This could range from a cozy bedroom to a clinical environment for medical play. The setting should evoke the desired atmosphere and align with the fantasy's theme.

3. **Character Development:** Develop characters that resonate with both partners. Consider their personalities, backgrounds, and motivations. This can deepen the emotional engagement and make the experience more immersive.

4. **Outline the Narrative:** Create a loose storyline that guides the role-play. This outline should include key plot points, emotional beats, and potential conflicts to enhance the drama and excitement.

5. **Incorporate Dialogue:** Dialogue is essential in role-playing scenarios. Craft lines that reflect the characters' desires, fears, and motivations. This dialogue can drive the narrative forward and create opportunities for intimacy.

6. **Establish Boundaries and Safewords:** Before engaging in role-play, partners should discuss and agree on boundaries and safewords. This ensures that both partners feel safe and respected throughout the experience.

Example Scenarios

To illustrate the concepts discussed, here are a few example scenarios that incorporate breeding fantasies:

- **The Fertile Encounter:** In this scenario, partners role-play a spontaneous encounter during a fertile window. The narrative could involve a romantic getaway where both partners express their desires to conceive, leading to passionate intimacy. The excitement of the moment, combined with the underlying theme of potential creation, enhances the erotic tension.

- **The Medical Examination:** This scenario involves one partner playing the role of a fertility specialist while the other takes on the role of a patient. The narrative could explore the dynamics of power and vulnerability, with the specialist providing intimate examinations and discussing the possibilities of conception. This scenario allows for the exploration of medical fetishization while maintaining a focus on consent and boundaries.

- **Postpartum Exploration:** After a pregnancy role-play, partners can explore the postpartum period. This scenario could involve one partner nurturing the other, focusing on themes of recovery, intimacy, and bonding. The narrative can highlight the emotional complexities of new parenthood, allowing for a deeper exploration of vulnerability and connection.

Psychological and Emotional Benefits

Engaging in erotic storytelling and role-playing scenarios offers numerous psychological and emotional benefits:

- **Enhanced Intimacy:** Sharing fantasies and engaging in role-play fosters a deeper emotional connection between partners. As they explore their desires together, they build trust and understanding.

- **Exploration of Identity:** Role-playing allows individuals to explore different aspects of their identities and desires. This exploration can lead to greater self-awareness and acceptance of one's fantasies.

- **Stress Relief:** Engaging in fantasy can serve as a form of escapism, providing a break from the stresses of daily life. The act of immersing oneself in a narrative can promote relaxation and enjoyment.

- **Communication Skills:** Discussing fantasies and engaging in role-play requires open communication. This practice can improve overall communication skills within the relationship, leading to a healthier dynamic.

Conclusion

Erotic storytelling and role-playing scenarios are invaluable tools for exploring breeding fantasies. By crafting narratives that resonate with personal desires and establishing safe, consensual environments, individuals and couples can deepen their intimacy and enrich their sexual experiences. As partners engage in these practices, they not only explore their fantasies but also strengthen their emotional bonds, paving the way for a more fulfilling and connected sexual relationship.

Erotic photography and videography

In the realm of breeding fantasy, erotic photography and videography serve as potent tools for expression, exploration, and enhancement of one's desires. These mediums allow individuals and couples to visually articulate their fantasies, providing a canvas where the intimate interplay of power dynamics, sensuality, and the allure of pregnancy can be vividly portrayed. This section delves into the theory behind erotic imagery, the practical considerations involved, and examples of how to effectively incorporate these elements into your breeding fantasy.

Theoretical Framework

The allure of erotic photography and videography lies in their capacity to capture and evoke emotions that words alone often fail to convey. Theories of eroticism suggest that visual stimuli can trigger physiological responses, such as increased heart rate and heightened arousal, which are essential in the context of breeding fantasies. According to [?], the concept of the "male gaze" plays a significant role in how erotic imagery is perceived; however, it is crucial to subvert this notion within the context of consensual breeding play, where both partners actively engage in the creation of their erotic narrative.

Additionally, the psychological impact of visual representation can enhance the experience of roleplay. As [?] posited, fantasies serve as a means of fulfilling desires that may be repressed or socially unacceptable. By capturing these fantasies through photography or videography, individuals can externalize and validate their desires, allowing for a deeper exploration of their identities and preferences.

Practical Considerations

When engaging in erotic photography and videography, several practical considerations must be addressed to ensure a positive and fulfilling experience:

1. **Consent and Boundaries**   Prior to any photographic or videographic session, it is imperative to establish clear consent and boundaries. Discuss what types of images or videos you are comfortable with, and ensure that both partners are on the same page regarding the content, context, and potential sharing of the material. This conversation should also encompass the use of safewords and check-ins during the shoot to maintain a supportive environment.

2. **Setting the Scene**   Creating an atmosphere conducive to erotic expression is vital. This can involve selecting a location that resonates with your fantasy, whether it be a private bedroom adorned with intimate lighting or a more adventurous outdoor setting. Consider the use of props that enhance the breeding theme, such as pregnancy pillows, maternity clothing, or other accessories that evoke the essence of your fantasy.

FANTASY ENHANCEMENT TECHNIQUES

3. **Equipment and Techniques** While professional equipment can elevate the quality of your images or videos, it is not a strict requirement. Modern smartphones often possess high-quality cameras capable of capturing intimate moments effectively. Experiment with different angles, lighting, and compositions to find what best represents your fantasy. Consider using techniques such as close-ups to emphasize intimacy or wide shots to capture the full scene.

4. **Editing and Enhancement** Post-production editing can significantly enhance the final product. Utilize editing software to adjust lighting, contrast, and color saturation, or to add filters that create a specific mood. However, it is essential to strike a balance; overly altering images can detract from the authenticity of the moment.

5. **Privacy and Security** Given the intimate nature of erotic photography and videography, privacy and security should be paramount. Discuss how the images will be stored and whether they will be shared with anyone outside your partnership. Consider using encrypted storage solutions or password-protected files to safeguard your content.

Examples of Incorporation

To effectively integrate erotic photography and videography into your breeding fantasy, consider the following examples:

1. **Documenting the Journey** Capture the various stages of your breeding fantasy, from the initial attempts at conception to the portrayal of pregnancy. This can include intimate moments of tenderness, playful exploration of fertility, or even staged scenarios that depict the excitement of trying to conceive.

2. **Role Reversal and Power Dynamics** Utilize photography to explore the dynamics of dominance and submission within your breeding fantasy. Consider staging scenarios where one partner takes on a more assertive role, while the other embodies submission, allowing the visual representation to enhance the emotional intensity of the experience.

3. **Fantasy Reenactments** Recreate specific scenes or fantasies that resonate with both partners. This could involve roleplaying a medical examination, a sensual encounter during the fertile window, or even the depiction of labor and birth.

These reenactments can be both playful and deeply intimate, allowing for a multifaceted exploration of your desires.

4. Community Engagement Engage with like-minded individuals by sharing your work within online communities or forums dedicated to breeding fantasies. This not only fosters a sense of belonging but also provides an opportunity for feedback and inspiration. Ensure that any shared content is consensual and respects the privacy of all involved.

Conclusion

Erotic photography and videography can significantly enhance the experience of breeding fantasy, providing a visual narrative that complements the emotional and psychological aspects of the roleplay. By understanding the theoretical underpinnings, addressing practical considerations, and creatively incorporating these mediums into your fantasy, individuals and couples can explore their desires in a safe, consensual, and fulfilling manner. As you embark on this journey, remember that the ultimate goal is to celebrate your fantasies and connect more deeply with your partner, embracing the beauty of erotic expression in all its forms.

Customizing sex toys and accessories

Customizing sex toys and accessories can significantly enhance the experience of breeding fantasy and erotic pregnancy play. Tailoring these items to fit personal preferences not only heightens arousal but also fosters a deeper connection to the fantasy. This section will explore various methods of customization, the psychological implications behind them, and practical examples to inspire creativity.

Understanding Personal Preferences

Before diving into customization, it is essential to understand individual preferences and desires. Each person's relationship with their body and sexuality is unique, influenced by factors such as past experiences, cultural backgrounds, and personal fantasies. Engaging in self-reflection or discussions with partners can help clarify what aspects of breeding fantasy resonate most strongly. This understanding serves as the foundation for effective customization.

Types of Customization

There are several ways to customize sex toys and accessories, which can range from aesthetic alterations to functional enhancements. Below are some common categories of customization:

- **Aesthetic Customization:** This involves altering the appearance of toys to align with the visual aspects of breeding fantasy. This can include:
  - *Color Choices:* Selecting colors that evoke the desired emotional response or match specific themes, such as soft pastels for a nurturing feel or darker shades for a more intense experience.
  - *Personalized Designs:* Engraving names, symbols, or meaningful phrases onto toys to create a sense of ownership and connection.
  - *Textured Surfaces:* Adding textures that mimic the sensations of pregnancy, such as rounded edges or soft, plush materials.

- **Functional Customization:** This focuses on enhancing the functionality of toys to better serve the needs of the user. Examples include:
  - *Adjustable Settings:* Opting for toys with customizable vibration patterns, intensities, and rhythms to cater to varying levels of arousal.
  - *Interchangeable Parts:* Choosing modular toys that allow users to swap out components, such as different attachments for dildos or vibrators, to explore various sensations.
  - *Size and Shape Modifications:* Selecting toys that can be molded or altered to fit anatomical preferences, ensuring comfort during use.

- **Incorporating Accessories:** Accessories can further enhance the breeding fantasy experience. Consider:
  - *Harnesses and Straps:* Utilizing harnesses to secure vibrators or dildos, allowing for hands-free play that can mimic the feeling of being penetrated or filled.
  - *Costumes and Lingerie:* Wearing outfits that align with the breeding fantasy, such as maternity-themed lingerie, can create a more immersive experience.
  - *Props and Tools:* Integrating items like pregnancy pillows or anatomical models can enrich the roleplay, providing visual and tactile stimulation.

Psychological Implications of Customization

The act of customizing sex toys and accessories can have profound psychological effects. Engaging in this process allows individuals to express their creativity and reinforce their connection to their fantasies. Customization can serve as a form of self-affirmation, validating one's desires and enhancing self-esteem. Furthermore, the anticipation of using customized toys can heighten arousal, turning the act of preparation into an integral part of the erotic experience.

Practical Examples of Customization

To illustrate the potential of customization, consider the following practical examples:

- **Customized Dildos:** A user may choose a dildo that mimics the shape and size they fantasize about. They might select a translucent material that allows for a view of internal mechanisms or even a glow-in-the-dark feature for added excitement during nighttime play.

- **Personalized Vibrators:** A couple could invest in a vibrator that can be programmed to respond to specific vocal commands, allowing for a more interactive experience. This customization not only enhances engagement but also reinforces the power dynamics present in breeding fantasies.

- **Themed Costumes:** A partner might create a costume that embodies the nurturing aspect of pregnancy, incorporating elements like flowing fabrics and soft textures. This costume can be paired with accessories like belly bands or faux baby bumps to enhance the visual representation of the fantasy.

Challenges in Customization

While customization can enhance the experience, it is essential to recognize potential challenges. These may include:

- **Safety Concerns:** Not all materials are safe for intimate use. When customizing, it is crucial to ensure that the materials are body-safe and non-toxic.

- **Cost Implications:** Customization may involve additional costs, which can be a barrier for some. It is important to balance desires with financial considerations.

- **Compatibility Issues:** When customizing toys, users must ensure that all components work well together. For example, a customized attachment may not fit all bases securely, leading to discomfort or safety risks during use.

Conclusion

Customizing sex toys and accessories can significantly enhance the experience of breeding fantasy and erotic pregnancy play. By understanding personal preferences, exploring various customization methods, and recognizing the psychological implications, individuals can create a more fulfilling and immersive experience. While challenges may arise, the benefits of customization can lead to greater intimacy and exploration within the realm of erotic fantasy. As you embark on this journey, remember that the ultimate goal is to create a safe, consensual, and pleasurable experience that resonates with your desires.

Incorporating elements of pregnancy fetish into fashion

Fashion is not merely a means of self-expression; it serves as a powerful medium through which individuals can communicate their desires, fantasies, and identities. In the realm of breeding fantasy and pregnancy fetish, the incorporation of specific elements into fashion can enhance the experience, allowing individuals to embody their fantasies in a tangible way. This section explores how to incorporate pregnancy fetish elements into fashion, addressing theory, potential challenges, and practical examples.

Theoretical Framework

The intersection of fashion and fetishism can be understood through several theoretical lenses, including psychoanalytic theory, gender studies, and semiotics. Psychoanalytic theory posits that clothing can serve as a projection of inner desires and fantasies. The act of dressing in a way that emphasizes or mimics pregnancy can evoke feelings of empowerment, submission, or nurturing, depending on the individual's psychological orientation towards their fantasy.

From a gender studies perspective, fashion is a site of both conformity and rebellion. By integrating elements of pregnancy fetish into everyday attire, individuals can challenge societal norms surrounding femininity, motherhood, and sexuality. This subversion allows for a redefinition of what it means to embody these roles, creating a space where traditional boundaries are blurred.

Semiotics, the study of signs and symbols, plays a critical role in understanding how fashion communicates meaning. The garments worn can symbolize fertility, femininity, and sensuality, while also serving as markers of identity within the fetish community. The colors, textures, and styles chosen can convey a range of emotions and messages, making fashion a rich language for expressing breeding fantasies.

Challenges and Considerations

Incorporating pregnancy fetish elements into fashion is not without its challenges. Societal stigma surrounding pregnancy and sexuality can lead to misunderstandings or negative judgments. It is essential to consider the context in which these fashion choices are made. For instance, wearing clothing that emphasizes pregnancy in a professional setting may provoke discomfort or backlash from colleagues.

Additionally, the emotional implications of embodying a pregnancy fantasy through fashion must be addressed. Some individuals may experience feelings of vulnerability, anxiety, or even shame when wearing garments that signify pregnancy. Establishing a supportive environment and engaging in open communication with partners can mitigate these feelings and enhance the overall experience.

Practical Examples

To effectively incorporate elements of pregnancy fetish into fashion, individuals can explore various styles, materials, and accessories. Below are several practical examples:

- **Maternity-Inspired Clothing:** Emphasizing the silhouette of pregnancy can be achieved through the use of flowy dresses, high-waisted skirts, and tops with empire waists. These styles can evoke a sense of nurturing and femininity while allowing for comfort and ease of movement.

- **Color Palette:** Soft pastel colors, such as baby blue, pink, and lavender, can evoke a sense of innocence and playfulness. In contrast, deeper shades like burgundy or forest green can convey a more sensual and mature interpretation of pregnancy. The choice of color can significantly impact the emotional tone of the outfit.

- **Textures and Fabrics:** Incorporating fabrics that mimic the feel of pregnancy, such as stretchy materials or soft knits, can enhance the experience. Latex, leather, or other fetish materials can also be used to create a more daring and provocative look, appealing to those who enjoy the intersection of pregnancy and BDSM aesthetics.

- **Accessories:** Accessories play a crucial role in completing the look. Items such as belly bands, faux baby bumps, or even jewelry that symbolizes fertility (like pendants shaped like eggs or wombs) can add depth to the outfit. Additionally, incorporating elements like lace or ribbons can enhance the sensuality of the attire.

- **Footwear:** The choice of footwear can also impact the overall aesthetic. High heels can elevate the outfit and create a more dominant presence, while flats or sandals may evoke a more nurturing and relaxed vibe. The balance between comfort and allure is crucial in this context.

- **Layering:** Experimenting with layering can create a dynamic look that allows for versatility. For example, pairing a fitted top with a flowing cardigan can highlight the pregnancy silhouette while providing options for revealing or concealing aspects of the outfit based on the scenario.

Creating a Personal Style

The key to successfully incorporating pregnancy fetish elements into fashion lies in personal expression and comfort. Each individual should feel empowered to create a style that resonates with their unique desires and fantasies. This may involve experimenting with different combinations of clothing, accessories, and styles to discover what feels most authentic and enjoyable.

Engaging with online communities and forums dedicated to pregnancy fetish and kink can also provide inspiration and support. Sharing ideas, outfits, and experiences can foster a sense of belonging and help individuals navigate the complexities of integrating these elements into their personal fashion.

Conclusion

Incorporating elements of pregnancy fetish into fashion is a powerful way to express desires and explore identities. By understanding the theoretical underpinnings, addressing potential challenges, and embracing practical examples, individuals can create a personal style that enhances their breeding fantasy. Ultimately, fashion becomes a canvas for self-exploration, allowing individuals to embody their fantasies with confidence and creativity.

Creating personalized scripts and fantasies

Creating personalized scripts and fantasies is an essential aspect of engaging in breeding fantasy and erotic pregnancy play. This process allows individuals and couples to tailor their experiences to align with their desires, boundaries, and emotional needs. By developing a script, participants can explore their fantasies in a structured manner, ensuring that the experience is both enjoyable and consensual.

Theoretical Framework

To understand the significance of personalized scripts, we can draw upon several theoretical frameworks:

- **Psychological Safety:** The concept of psychological safety, as described by Edmondson (1999), emphasizes the importance of creating an environment where individuals feel safe to express their thoughts and feelings without fear of judgment. Personalized scripts can enhance this safety by providing a clear structure for exploration.

- **Narrative Therapy:** According to White and Epston (1990), narrative therapy posits that individuals construct their identities through stories. By crafting personalized scripts, participants can actively shape their narratives, allowing for greater agency and self-exploration.

- **Role Theory:** Role theory, as proposed by Biddle (1986), suggests that individuals perform roles based on social expectations. In the context of breeding fantasy, scripts allow participants to define their roles, enhancing the immersive experience of roleplay.

Steps to Create a Personalized Script

Creating a personalized script involves several steps that ensure the fantasy aligns with the desires and boundaries of all participants:

1. **Identify Desires and Boundaries:** Begin by discussing what each participant hopes to explore within the breeding fantasy. This may include specific scenarios, emotional themes, and physical actions. It is crucial to establish boundaries to avoid discomfort or emotional distress.

2. **Choose a Scenario:** Select a scenario that resonates with both participants. Some popular scenarios include natural conception, fertility clinics, or even fantastical elements like time travel or alternate realities. The chosen scenario should evoke excitement and align with the participants' interests.

3. **Outline Key Elements:** Create an outline that includes key elements of the script, such as characters, setting, dialogue, and actions. This outline serves as a roadmap for the roleplay, ensuring that both participants remain engaged and focused.

4. **Incorporate Dialogue:** Writing dialogue can enhance the authenticity of the roleplay. Consider how characters would realistically communicate in the chosen scenario. Use language that reflects the emotional tone of the fantasy, whether it be tender, playful, or intense.

5. **Plan for Emotional Dynamics:** Recognize that breeding fantasy often involves complex emotional dynamics. Consider how power exchange, vulnerability, and intimacy will play out within the script. Plan for moments of connection and potential conflict, allowing for a richer narrative.

6. **Review and Revise:** Once the initial script is drafted, review it together. Discuss any aspects that may need adjustment to better fit comfort levels or desires. This collaborative revision process fosters communication and strengthens trust.

7. **Practice and Roleplay:** Engage in the roleplay, using the script as a guide. Allow for spontaneity and improvisation, as these elements can lead to unexpected and enjoyable moments. After the roleplay, discuss the experience, noting what worked well and what could be improved for future sessions.

Examples of Personalized Scripts

Here are a few examples of personalized scripts that can serve as inspiration:

- **Natural Conception Scenario:**

    Setting: A cozy bedroom, soft lighting. The couple is preparing for a romantic evening, discussing their desire to start a family.
    Dialogue:

    Partner A: "I've been thinking about how amazing it would be to create something together. Just imagine... a little version of us."
    Partner B: "I know! The thought of you carrying our child makes me feel so connected to you."

- Fertility Clinic Roleplay:

    Setting: A clinical environment, complete with medical props. The couple is roleplaying a visit to a fertility specialist.

    Dialogue:

    Doctor: "Let's discuss your options for starting a family. How do you both feel about artificial insemination?"
    Partner A: "We are excited but also nervous. It's a big step for us."
    Partner B: "I trust you completely. Whatever we choose, I want to do it together."

- Fantasy Insemination:

    Setting: A magical realm where conception can occur through enchanted rituals.

    Dialogue:

    Partner A: "In this world, we can create life with a single touch. Are you ready to embrace the magic?"
    Partner B: "Yes! Let's make our dreams come true together, surrounded by the stars."

Addressing Potential Problems

While creating personalized scripts can enhance the experience, it is essential to acknowledge potential problems that may arise:

- **Miscommunication:** Clear communication is vital to avoid misunderstandings. Regular check-ins before and during the roleplay can help ensure that both participants feel comfortable and engaged.

- **Emotional Triggers:** Some elements of breeding fantasy may evoke strong emotions. It is important to discuss potential triggers beforehand and establish a plan for addressing them during the roleplay.

- **Rigid Scripts:** While scripts provide structure, they should not be overly rigid. Allowing for improvisation can lead to a more authentic and enjoyable experience.

- **Post-Roleplay Reflection:** After the roleplay, it is crucial to engage in a debriefing session. Discuss what aspects were enjoyable, what could be improved, and any emotions that arose during the experience. This reflection fosters growth and understanding.

Conclusion

Creating personalized scripts and fantasies is a powerful tool for exploring breeding fantasy and erotic pregnancy play. By engaging in this process, participants can enhance their emotional connection, navigate complex dynamics, and foster a safe space for exploration. With clear communication, mutual consent, and a willingness to adapt, personalized scripts can transform fantasies into deeply intimate experiences that resonate long after the roleplay has concluded.

Joining Online Communities and Forums

In today's digital age, online communities and forums serve as essential platforms for individuals exploring their breeding fantasies and engaging in erotic pregnancy play. These virtual spaces provide a unique opportunity for individuals to connect with like-minded people, share experiences, and seek advice in a safe environment. This section delves into the benefits, challenges, and best practices for joining online communities and forums related to breeding fantasies.

Benefits of Online Communities

Connection and Support One of the primary advantages of joining online communities is the ability to connect with others who share similar interests. For many, breeding fantasies can be a source of shame or secrecy in their offline lives. Online forums provide a non-judgmental space where individuals can express their desires, seek validation, and find emotional support. This sense of belonging can significantly enhance one's self-acceptance and confidence in exploring their fantasies.

Sharing Knowledge and Resources Online communities often serve as repositories of knowledge, where members share resources, articles, and personal experiences related to breeding play. This exchange of information can be invaluable for newcomers seeking to understand the intricacies of their fantasies. For instance, forums might discuss safe practices for roleplaying, effective communication strategies with partners, or personal anecdotes that help demystify the experience of pregnancy play.

Diverse Perspectives Engaging with a wide range of individuals allows members to gain insights from various perspectives. Different cultural backgrounds, experiences, and interpretations of breeding fantasies can enrich one's understanding and appreciation of the fetish. This diversity fosters a more inclusive environment where individuals can explore the many facets of their desires without fear of judgment.

Challenges of Online Communities

Privacy and Anonymity Concerns While online communities can offer a sense of anonymity, they also pose risks regarding privacy. Users must be vigilant about protecting their personal information and ensuring that their engagement in these communities does not lead to unwanted exposure. It is crucial to use pseudonyms and avoid sharing identifiable details to maintain privacy.

Misinformation and Misunderstanding The open nature of online forums means that not all information shared is accurate or helpful. Members may encounter misinformation regarding safe practices, consent, or the psychological aspects of breeding play. It is essential to approach online discussions critically and verify information through reputable sources or expert opinions.

Toxicity and Judgment Despite the potential for supportive environments, some online communities can harbor toxic behavior, including judgment, shaming, or harassment. Members should be prepared to navigate these challenges and prioritize their mental well-being. Recognizing red flags, such as aggressive behavior or dismissive attitudes, is vital for maintaining a positive experience.

Best Practices for Joining Online Communities

Choosing the Right Community When seeking online communities, it is essential to find spaces that align with one's interests and values. Look for forums that emphasize consent, respect, and inclusivity. Reading community guidelines and observing interactions before joining can help identify whether a particular space is welcoming and supportive.

Engaging Respectfully Active participation in online communities involves engaging respectfully with others. This means being open to different viewpoints, offering support, and adhering to community guidelines. Practicing empathy and understanding fosters a positive environment and encourages others to share their experiences.

Setting Boundaries While online communities can be a source of support, it is crucial to establish personal boundaries. Members should feel empowered to disengage from discussions that make them uncomfortable or violate their boundaries. Setting limits on the information shared and the interactions pursued can help maintain a healthy balance between engagement and personal safety.

Utilizing Resources Wisely Many online communities offer resources such as articles, guides, or webinars. Members should take advantage of these resources to enhance their understanding of breeding fantasies. Engaging with educational content can empower individuals to explore their desires safely and responsibly.

Examples of Online Communities

FetLife FetLife is one of the largest social networking platforms for individuals with various fetishes, including breeding fantasies. Users can create profiles, join groups, and participate in discussions that cater to their specific interests. The platform emphasizes consent and safe practices, making it a valuable resource for those exploring breeding play.

Reddit Subreddits such as /r/Breeding and /r/BreedingFetish provide spaces for individuals to share their experiences, seek advice, and discuss fantasies related to breeding. Reddit's upvote and downvote system helps highlight valuable content, allowing users to engage with the most relevant discussions.

Discord Servers Many Discord servers focus on niche interests, including breeding fantasies. These servers offer real-time chat and voice communication, allowing for more dynamic interactions. Members can join discussions, share resources, and participate in events or workshops tailored to their interests.

Conclusion

Joining online communities and forums dedicated to breeding fantasies can be a transformative experience for individuals seeking connection, knowledge, and support. By navigating these spaces thoughtfully, members can enhance their understanding of their desires while fostering a sense of belonging within a diverse and inclusive environment. As with any exploration of erotic interests, prioritizing consent, safety, and personal well-being is paramount for a fulfilling experience in the realm of breeding fantasy.

Attending events and workshops

Attending events and workshops dedicated to breeding fantasies and erotic pregnancy play can be an enriching experience for those interested in exploring their desires in a safe and consensual environment. These gatherings often provide opportunities for education, community building, and practical engagement with various aspects of breeding fantasy.

Types of Events and Workshops

Events and workshops can vary widely in focus and format. Some may be structured around educational seminars, while others may include hands-on activities, role-playing scenarios, or discussion groups. Common types of events include:

- **Educational Workshops:** These sessions often feature experts discussing topics such as safe practices, psychological aspects of breeding play, and effective communication strategies. Participants can gain valuable insights into their fantasies and learn how to navigate them responsibly.

- **Roleplay Events:** These gatherings encourage participants to engage in role-playing scenarios in a controlled setting. They often provide a safe space to explore various breeding fantasies with like-minded individuals, fostering a sense of community and support.

- **Conventions and Festivals:** Larger events may combine multiple workshops, presentations, and social activities. These conventions often feature vendors, performances, and opportunities to connect with others who share similar interests in breeding and pregnancy play.

- **Support Groups:** Some workshops focus on the emotional and psychological aspects of breeding fantasies, providing a space for individuals to share experiences, discuss challenges, and offer support to one another.

Benefits of Attending

The benefits of attending events and workshops centered on breeding fantasy are numerous:

- **Education and Awareness:** Participants can deepen their understanding of breeding fantasies, learning about the psychological, emotional, and physical aspects associated with them. This knowledge can empower individuals to explore their desires more confidently and safely.

- **Community Building:** Engaging with others who share similar interests fosters a sense of belonging and reduces feelings of isolation. Building connections within the community can lead to lasting friendships and support networks.

- **Skill Development:** Workshops often provide practical skills that can enhance role-playing experiences. From negotiating boundaries to exploring techniques for safe play, participants can leave with new tools for engaging in their fantasies.

- **Safe Exploration:** Events typically prioritize consent and safety, allowing individuals to explore their fantasies in a controlled environment. This structure can help mitigate risks and enhance the overall experience.

Challenges and Considerations

While attending events and workshops can be beneficial, there are challenges and considerations to keep in mind:

- **Personal Comfort Levels:** Not all individuals may feel comfortable engaging in public displays of their breeding fantasies. It is essential to assess one's comfort level and choose events that align with personal boundaries.

- **Consent and Boundaries:** Clear communication about consent and boundaries is crucial in any group setting. Participants should be proactive in discussing their limits and ensuring that others respect them.

- **Social Stigma:** Despite increasing acceptance of diverse sexualities, some individuals may still face judgment or stigma. It is important to prepare for potential societal backlash and to have strategies in place for handling negative reactions.

- **Cost and Accessibility:** Some events may have associated costs, such as registration fees or travel expenses. It is important to consider financial implications and seek out events that fit within one's budget.

Finding Events and Workshops

To locate relevant events and workshops, consider the following strategies:

- **Online Communities:** Join online forums, social media groups, or websites dedicated to breeding fantasies and erotic roleplay. These platforms often share information about upcoming events and workshops.

- **Local Kink and BDSM Groups:** Many cities have local kink or BDSM organizations that host events. Connecting with these groups can provide access to a variety of workshops and gatherings focused on breeding and pregnancy play.

- **Conventions and Expos:** Attend larger conventions that focus on sexuality, kink, or alternative lifestyles. These events often feature a wide range of workshops and presentations on various topics, including breeding fantasies.

- **Word of Mouth:** Networking within the community can lead to discovering events that may not be widely advertised. Engaging in conversations with others can provide valuable insights and recommendations.

Conclusion

Attending events and workshops focused on breeding fantasies and erotic pregnancy play can significantly enhance one's understanding and enjoyment of these desires. By engaging with knowledgeable facilitators and connecting with like-minded individuals, participants can explore their fantasies in a safe and supportive environment. However, it is essential to approach these experiences with an awareness of personal boundaries, consent, and the potential challenges that may arise. Ultimately, the journey into breeding fantasy can lead to profound self-discovery and deeper connections with oneself and others.

Managing the balance between reality and fantasy

In the realm of breeding fantasy and erotic pregnancy play, the line between reality and fantasy can often blur, creating a complex landscape that requires careful navigation. It is essential to maintain a healthy balance to ensure that the experiences remain pleasurable and fulfilling without crossing into harmful territory. This section explores the theoretical frameworks, potential problems, and practical examples to aid individuals and couples in managing this balance.

Theoretical Frameworks

The dynamics of fantasy and reality can be understood through several psychological theories. One relevant concept is **escapism**, which refers to the tendency to seek distraction and relief from unpleasant realities through fantasy. While escapism can provide a temporary reprieve, it is crucial to recognize when it becomes a coping mechanism that may lead to avoidance of real-life responsibilities or issues.

Another important theory is **psychological projection**, where individuals project their desires and fears onto their fantasies. In breeding fantasy, this may manifest as a desire for control, intimacy, or even a longing for nurturing relationships. Understanding these projections can help individuals discern which elements of their fantasies are rooted in genuine desires versus those that may stem from unresolved emotional conflicts.

Problems of Imbalance

The imbalance between reality and fantasy can lead to several issues, including:

- **Disillusionment:** When fantasies are pursued without acknowledging their fictional nature, individuals may face disappointment when reality does not align with their expectations. For instance, a couple may engage in roleplay that feels intensely fulfilling, only to struggle with intimacy in their everyday relationship.

- **Dependency:** An over-reliance on fantasy can lead to neglecting real-world relationships and responsibilities. If one partner becomes increasingly absorbed in breeding fantasies, the other may feel isolated or unvalued, leading to resentment and conflict.

- **Confusion of Roles:** In roleplay scenarios, the participants may find it challenging to separate their real identities from their fantasy personas. This confusion can lead to misunderstandings and emotional distress, particularly if the roleplay involves power dynamics that are not present in the everyday relationship.

Practical Strategies for Balance

To maintain a healthy balance between reality and fantasy, consider the following strategies:

BEYOND THE BEDROOM: INTEGRATING BREEDING FANTASY INTO DAILY LIFE

1. **Regular Check-Ins:** Establish a routine of open communication where both partners can express their feelings about the fantasy and its impact on their relationship. This practice can help identify any discomfort or disconnection that may arise.

2. **Set Boundaries:** Clearly define the limits of your roleplay. This includes discussing what elements of the fantasy are acceptable and which are not. For example, while exploring the thrill of insemination may be exciting, it's vital to agree on what happens if the fantasy starts to feel too real or uncomfortable.

3. **Incorporate Reality into Fantasy:** Blend elements of your real-life relationship into the fantasy scenarios. This can enhance intimacy and ensure that both partners feel connected. For instance, discussing how the fantasy of pregnancy might influence your real-life plans for family can create a bridge between the two worlds.

4. **Engage in Aftercare:** After roleplay sessions, engage in aftercare practices to reinforce emotional safety and connection. This can include cuddling, discussing what worked well, and addressing any feelings that emerged during the play.

5. **Seek Professional Guidance:** If navigating the balance proves challenging, consider consulting with a therapist who specializes in sexual health or relationship dynamics. They can provide tailored strategies and support to help both partners explore their fantasies healthily and constructively.

Examples of Balance in Action

Consider a couple, Alex and Jamie, who enjoy exploring breeding fantasies. They begin by discussing their desires and establishing clear boundaries. During their roleplay, they incorporate real-life elements, such as their shared love for cooking, by roleplaying a scenario where they prepare a meal together while discussing their fantasy.

After each session, they prioritize aftercare, taking time to cuddle and share their feelings about the experience. They regularly check in with each other, ensuring that neither feels overwhelmed or disconnected from their reality. This approach allows them to enjoy their fantasies while maintaining a strong, healthy relationship grounded in mutual respect and understanding.

Conclusion

Managing the balance between reality and fantasy in breeding play requires ongoing communication, self-awareness, and a commitment to emotional safety. By employing theoretical insights and practical strategies, individuals and couples can explore their desires while ensuring that their real-life relationships remain fulfilling and supportive. Ultimately, the goal is to create a space where fantasy can enrich reality without overshadowing it, allowing for an intimate exploration of desires that honors both partners' needs and boundaries.

Ethical Considerations and Conclusion

Consent and Boundaries Revisited

Reevaluating boundaries and limits

In the realm of breeding fantasy and erotic roleplay, the concept of boundaries is not merely a guideline but a vital framework for safe exploration. As desires evolve and experiences deepen, it becomes essential to periodically reevaluate these boundaries to ensure that both partners feel secure, respected, and fulfilled in their shared fantasies. This section will explore the significance of reassessing limits, highlight potential challenges, and provide practical strategies for navigating this complex aspect of intimate relationships.

The Importance of Reevaluation

Reevaluation of boundaries serves several critical functions:

- **Adaptation to Change:** As individuals grow and change, so too may their desires and comfort levels. What once felt exhilarating might become overwhelming or vice versa. Regular check-ins allow partners to adapt their roleplay to reflect these shifts.

- **Enhancing Trust:** Open discussions about boundaries foster an environment of trust. When partners know they can voice their needs and concerns without fear of judgment, it strengthens their emotional connection.

- **Preventing Misunderstandings:** Clear communication reduces the risk of misinterpretations that could lead to discomfort or harm during roleplay.

Regularly revisiting boundaries ensures that both partners are on the same page.

Challenges in Reevaluating Boundaries

Despite the benefits, partners may encounter several challenges when attempting to reevaluate boundaries:

- **Fear of Rejection:** One partner may hesitate to express their changing needs due to fear that the other will reject them or the fantasy altogether. This fear can stifle open communication and lead to resentment.

- **Power Dynamics:** In scenarios involving power exchange, the dominant partner may unintentionally impose their desires on the submissive partner, making it difficult for the latter to voice their limits. This can create an imbalance that undermines the safety of the roleplay.

- **Guilt and Shame:** Individuals may feel guilty or ashamed for wanting to change established boundaries, especially if they perceive their desires as taboo or inappropriate. These feelings can lead to internal conflict and hinder honest discussions.

Strategies for Effective Reevaluation

To effectively navigate the reevaluation of boundaries, consider the following strategies:

- **Scheduled Check-Ins:** Establish regular intervals for discussing boundaries, such as after a roleplay session or weekly. This creates a safe space for both partners to express their feelings and reassess limits without the pressure of immediate context.

- **Utilizing "I" Statements:** Encourage the use of "I" statements to express feelings and desires. For example, "I feel uncomfortable when…" rather than "You make me feel uncomfortable." This approach minimizes defensiveness and promotes understanding.

- **Roleplay Scenarios for Exploration:** Consider incorporating roleplay scenarios specifically designed to explore boundaries. For instance, a "negotiation" scene can allow partners to act out discussions about limits in a playful context, helping to alleviate tension.

- **Documentation of Limits:** Keeping a written record of agreed-upon boundaries can serve as a reference point for both partners. This documentation can be revisited during check-ins to facilitate discussions about changes.

- **Encouraging Openness:** Foster an atmosphere of openness where both partners feel safe to express their evolving desires. Reassure each other that it is acceptable to change limits without fear of judgment or rejection.

- **Professional Guidance:** If challenges persist, consider seeking the guidance of a therapist or counselor experienced in BDSM and kink dynamics. Professional support can provide tools and techniques for navigating complex emotional landscapes.

Examples of Boundary Reevaluation in Practice

To illustrate the process of boundary reevaluation, consider the following examples:

- **Example 1:** A couple has established a boundary around the types of roleplay scenarios they engage in, with one partner feeling uncomfortable with the idea of medical play. After several months, the partner who initially set this boundary begins to feel curious about exploring medical themes. During a scheduled check-in, they express this curiosity, leading to a constructive conversation about potential scenarios that could feel safe and exciting for both.

- **Example 2:** In a dominant/submissive dynamic, the submissive partner has previously agreed to a specific set of limits. Over time, they find that certain aspects of the roleplay no longer resonate with them. They approach their dominant partner during a check-in, using "I" statements to express their feelings. The dominant partner listens and acknowledges the submissive's needs, leading to a revised agreement that respects the evolving dynamics of their relationship.

- **Example 3:** A couple engaged in breeding fantasy roleplay has established a boundary regarding the use of certain language that one partner finds triggering. After a few sessions, the partner who set this limit realizes they want to explore that language in a safe context. They bring this up during a check-in, discussing how they can introduce it gradually while ensuring that both partners feel secure.

Conclusion

Reevaluating boundaries and limits is a crucial aspect of engaging in breeding fantasy and erotic roleplay. It requires ongoing communication, trust, and a willingness to adapt as desires evolve. By acknowledging the challenges, employing effective strategies, and drawing on real-life examples, partners can create a safe and fulfilling space for exploration. Ultimately, the goal is to ensure that both individuals feel empowered to express their needs and desires, fostering a deeper connection and enhancing the overall experience of their intimate journey together.

Prioritizing consent and communication

In the realm of erotic roleplay, particularly within the context of breeding fantasies, the principles of consent and communication are paramount. Consent is not merely a checkbox; it is a dynamic, ongoing dialogue that evolves throughout the experience. This section delves into the critical aspects of prioritizing consent and fostering effective communication, ensuring a safe and enjoyable exploration of breeding fantasies.

The Foundation of Consent

Consent is the cornerstone of any intimate interaction. In the context of breeding fantasies, it takes on additional layers of complexity due to the sensitive nature of the themes involved. The foundational elements of consent include:

- **Informed Consent:** All parties involved must have a clear understanding of the activities they are consenting to. This includes discussing the specifics of the roleplay scenario, boundaries, and any potential risks involved. For example, if a couple is roleplaying a scenario involving artificial insemination, both partners should discuss what that entails, including emotional and physical implications.

- **Voluntary Consent:** Consent must be given freely, without coercion or pressure. This means that all parties should feel empowered to express their desires and limitations without fear of judgment or retaliation. For instance, if one partner expresses discomfort with a particular aspect of the roleplay, their feelings should be respected without any attempts to persuade them otherwise.

- **Revocable Consent:** Consent can be withdrawn at any time. It is essential to create an environment where all participants feel safe to change their minds.

For example, during a roleplay session, if a participant feels overwhelmed or uncomfortable, they should be able to use a safeword or signal to halt the activity immediately.

Communication Techniques

Effective communication is integral to navigating the complexities of breeding fantasies. Here are several techniques to enhance communication between partners:

- **Pre-Play Discussions:** Before engaging in any roleplay, partners should have an open and honest conversation about their interests, boundaries, and any concerns. This discussion should cover the specifics of the breeding fantasy, including any particular scenarios or dynamics that excite them. For instance, a couple might discuss their feelings about exploring themes of dominance and submission within the context of breeding.

- **Active Listening:** Partners should practice active listening, which involves fully concentrating on what the other person is saying, understanding their message, responding thoughtfully, and remembering key points. This can be crucial when discussing sensitive topics like emotional triggers or past experiences that may influence the roleplay.

- **Check-Ins:** Regular check-ins during the roleplay can help ensure that all parties are comfortable and enjoying the experience. Simple questions like, "How are you feeling?" or "Is this still okay for you?" can promote a sense of safety and awareness. For example, during a scene, one partner might pause to ask if the other is still comfortable with the direction the roleplay is taking.

- **Post-Play Debriefing:** After the roleplay, it is beneficial to engage in a debriefing session. This allows partners to discuss what worked well, what could be improved, and any feelings that arose during the experience. For instance, one partner might express that they felt a strong emotional response during a particular scene, prompting a deeper conversation about its impact.

Addressing Common Challenges

Despite the best intentions, challenges may arise in prioritizing consent and communication. Here are some common issues and strategies to address them:

- **Miscommunication:** Misunderstandings can occur, especially when discussing sensitive topics. To mitigate this, partners should clarify any ambiguous statements and reiterate their understanding of the agreed-upon boundaries. Using clear language and avoiding euphemisms can help ensure that both partners are on the same page.

- **Fear of Judgment:** Participants may hesitate to express their true desires due to fear of being judged. Creating a non-judgmental space is essential. Partners should reassure each other that all fantasies are valid and that honesty is crucial for a fulfilling experience. For example, sharing a fantasy about a taboo scenario should be met with curiosity rather than criticism.

- **Power Imbalances:** In scenarios involving dominant and submissive roles, power dynamics can complicate consent. It is vital to establish clear boundaries and ensure that both partners feel empowered to voice their needs. Regular check-ins can help maintain an equilibrium of power and ensure that the submissive partner feels safe and respected.

- **Emotional Triggers:** Breeding fantasies can evoke strong emotions, and triggers may arise unexpectedly. It is essential to discuss potential triggers beforehand and establish a plan for addressing them if they occur. For instance, if one partner has experienced pregnancy loss, they should communicate this to their partner, who can then be mindful of how certain scenarios might affect them.

Real-Life Example

Consider a couple, Alex and Jamie, who are exploring breeding fantasies. Before engaging in their roleplay, they sit down to discuss their interests. Jamie expresses a desire to explore the theme of artificial insemination, while Alex is intrigued by the idea of natural conception. They agree to incorporate both elements into their roleplay, ensuring that they communicate openly about their boundaries.

During their scene, Jamie begins to feel overwhelmed by the intensity of the roleplay. Remembering their pre-established safeword, they pause the activity and communicate their discomfort. Alex listens attentively, reassures Jamie, and they take a moment to recalibrate their scene, focusing on a softer, more intimate approach.

After the roleplay, they engage in a debriefing session, where they both share their feelings about the experience. Jamie expresses gratitude for Alex's understanding, while Alex appreciates Jamie's honesty. This open communication strengthens their bond and enhances their future roleplay experiences.

Conclusion

Prioritizing consent and communication is essential in the exploration of breeding fantasies. By establishing a foundation of informed, voluntary, and revocable consent, and employing effective communication techniques, partners can navigate the complexities of their desires safely and enjoyably. Addressing common challenges with empathy and understanding further reinforces the importance of these principles, ensuring that the exploration of breeding fantasies is a fulfilling and enriching experience for all involved.

Addressing power imbalances and coercion

In the realm of breeding fantasy and erotic roleplay, addressing power imbalances and coercion is paramount. Power dynamics are inherent in many sexual relationships, particularly in kink and fetish contexts. Understanding these dynamics is crucial for ensuring that all parties involved engage in consensual and fulfilling experiences. This section will delve into the theoretical underpinnings of power imbalances, the potential for coercion, and practical strategies for navigating these challenges.

Theoretical Framework

Power dynamics in relationships can be understood through various theoretical lenses, including *Foucault's theory of power* and *BDSM frameworks*. Michel Foucault posited that power is not merely held but is a relational phenomenon that circulates among individuals. In the context of breeding fantasy, power can manifest in several forms:

- **Physical Power:** The ability to exert physical control or dominance over a partner.

- **Emotional Power:** The capacity to influence a partner's feelings or emotional state, often through manipulation or coercion.

- **Social Power:** The impact of societal norms and expectations on individual desires and behaviors.

- **Economic Power:** The influence of financial resources on relationship dynamics, particularly in scenarios involving gifts, services, or financial dependency.

Identifying Coercion

Coercion can be subtle and may not always present as overt force. It can manifest in various ways, including:

- **Emotional Manipulation:** Using guilt or emotional distress to pressure a partner into participating in a fantasy.

- **Social Pressure:** Leveraging social dynamics or peer influence to coerce a partner into engaging in practices they are uncomfortable with.

- **Financial Dependency:** Exploiting economic imbalances, where one partner may feel obligated to comply due to financial reliance on the other.

To illustrate, consider a scenario where one partner expresses interest in breeding fantasies while the other is hesitant. If the interested partner responds with emotional guilt, suggesting that their relationship depends on the other's participation, this constitutes emotional manipulation and coercion.

Strategies for Addressing Power Imbalances

To foster a safe and consensual environment, individuals must actively work to recognize and address power imbalances. Here are several strategies:

- **Open Communication:** Establish a culture of transparency where both partners can express their desires, fears, and boundaries without fear of judgment or retribution. Utilizing *active listening* techniques can enhance understanding and empathy.

- **Negotiation:** Prior to engaging in breeding fantasies, partners should negotiate the specifics of their roleplay. This includes discussing desires, limits, and potential triggers. Documenting these agreements can help reinforce mutual understanding.

- **Safewords and Check-ins:** Implementing safewords allows partners to halt the roleplay if they feel uncomfortable or coerced. Regular check-ins during the experience can also provide opportunities for reassessment and adjustment of boundaries.

- **Educating on Consent:** Both partners should have a clear understanding of what constitutes consent and the importance of ongoing consent throughout the roleplay. This includes recognizing that consent can be revoked at any time and should be respected without question.

- **Power Exchange Dynamics:** If engaging in power exchange, it is essential to discuss the implications of this dynamic. Both partners should agree on how power will be exchanged and what safeguards are in place to prevent coercion.

- **Aftercare:** Aftercare is a crucial component of any BDSM or roleplay scenario, particularly when power dynamics are involved. It allows partners to reconnect, discuss their experiences, and ensure emotional well-being post-play.

Recognizing Red Flags

Being aware of red flags can help partners identify potential coercive dynamics early. Some common indicators include:

- One partner consistently dismisses the other's feelings or boundaries.

- There is a pattern of guilt-tripping or emotional manipulation.

- Disproportionate power dynamics, where one partner makes unilateral decisions without consulting the other.

- A lack of aftercare or emotional support post-roleplay.

Conclusion

Addressing power imbalances and coercion in breeding fantasy and erotic roleplay requires vigilance, open communication, and a commitment to mutual respect. By recognizing the complexities of power dynamics and implementing strategies to foster consent and safety, partners can explore their fantasies in a way that is fulfilling and empowering. Ultimately, the goal is to create a space where both partners feel valued, respected, and free to express their desires without fear of coercion or manipulation.

Handling conflicting desires and fantasies

Navigating the intricate landscape of sexual desires and fantasies can often feel like traversing a minefield, especially when conflicting desires arise within oneself or between partners. In the realm of breeding fantasy, where the stakes involve deeply personal emotions and societal taboos, managing these conflicts requires sensitivity, communication, and a keen understanding of the psychological underpinnings at play.

Understanding Conflicting Desires

Conflicting desires can manifest in various forms, such as a yearning for the thrill of breeding fantasies juxtaposed with fears of actual pregnancy, or a partner's enthusiasm for roleplay clashing with another's discomfort regarding the implications of that fantasy. The psychological theory of *cognitive dissonance* (Festinger, 1957) explains how individuals experience mental discomfort when holding two or more contradictory beliefs, values, or desires. This discomfort can lead to anxiety, confusion, and avoidance behaviors, which can complicate intimate relationships.

To illustrate, consider a couple where one partner is excited about engaging in breeding fantasies, while the other feels apprehensive due to personal experiences or societal pressures. The partner who embraces the fantasy may feel rejected or misunderstood, while the apprehensive partner may experience guilt for not fully participating. This dynamic can create a rift that, if left unaddressed, could lead to resentment or withdrawal.

The Importance of Open Communication

The cornerstone of resolving conflicting desires lies in open communication. Establishing a safe space for dialogue allows partners to express their feelings without fear of judgment. Active listening is crucial; it involves not only hearing the words spoken but also understanding the emotions and motivations behind them.

$$\text{Active Listening} = \text{Empathy} + \text{Validation} + \text{Reflection} \qquad (18)$$

For instance, one partner might say, "I feel anxious about exploring breeding fantasies because I worry about the reality of pregnancy." The other partner can respond with empathy: "I understand that this is a significant concern for you, and I appreciate you sharing it with me." This approach fosters a sense of safety and encourages further exploration of each partner's feelings.

Negotiating Boundaries and Compromises

Once the conflicting desires are articulated, the next step is to negotiate boundaries and find compromises that honor both partners' needs. This process may involve exploring alternative scenarios that align more closely with each person's comfort levels. For example, if one partner is uncomfortable with the idea of actual pregnancy, they might agree to roleplay scenarios that emphasize the fantasy aspect without the implication of real-life consequences, such as focusing on the excitement of conception without the physicality of pregnancy.

Utilizing the concept of *consensual non-monogamy* (Barker, 2005), partners can also explore the possibility of seeking fulfillment outside the primary relationship, provided that both parties consent and communicate openly about their experiences. This approach can alleviate pressure and allow each partner to explore their desires in a manner that feels safe and respectful.

Addressing Emotional Triggers

Conflicting desires can often be rooted in deeper emotional triggers. For instance, a partner may have past trauma related to pregnancy or childbirth, leading to heightened anxiety when confronted with breeding fantasies. Recognizing these triggers is essential for fostering understanding and compassion within the relationship.

Employing techniques from *trauma-informed care* can be beneficial in these situations. This approach emphasizes the importance of creating a safe environment, recognizing the impact of trauma, and integrating this understanding into communication and roleplay. For example, if a partner expresses discomfort, it is vital to pause the roleplay and engage in a check-in, allowing space for the partner to articulate their feelings and re-establish boundaries.

Utilizing Professional Support

In cases where conflicting desires lead to significant distress or relationship strain, seeking professional support from a therapist or counselor specializing in sexual health and relationships can be invaluable. Professionals can provide a neutral space for partners to explore their desires, facilitate communication, and help navigate the complexities of their fantasies.

Therapists may employ techniques such as *emotionally focused therapy* (Johnson, 2004), which focuses on identifying and transforming negative patterns of interaction between partners, fostering emotional connection, and enhancing intimacy. By working through these dynamics with a trained professional, partners can gain insights into their desires and develop healthier communication strategies.

Fostering Personal Growth and Self-Discovery

Ultimately, handling conflicting desires and fantasies can lead to profound personal growth and self-discovery. Engaging in self-reflection allows individuals to explore the roots of their desires and the underlying emotions that shape them. Journaling, for instance, can be a powerful tool for unpacking feelings related to breeding fantasies, helping individuals articulate their needs and fears.

Furthermore, attending workshops or joining support groups focused on sexual exploration can provide valuable insights and foster a sense of community. Sharing experiences with others who navigate similar desires can normalize the complexities of sexual fantasies and reinforce the notion that conflict is a natural part of human sexuality.

Conclusion

In conclusion, handling conflicting desires and fantasies within the context of breeding play requires a multifaceted approach that prioritizes communication, empathy, and understanding. By recognizing the psychological dimensions of these conflicts, partners can foster a deeper connection, navigate their desires with respect, and ultimately enhance their intimate experiences. Embracing the complexities of sexual fantasies can lead to enriched relationships and a more profound understanding of oneself and one's partner.

Recognizing and addressing red flags

In the realm of breeding fantasy and erotic roleplay, it is crucial to maintain a vigilant awareness of potential red flags that may indicate unhealthy dynamics or risks to the well-being of those involved. Recognizing these warning signs is essential for fostering a safe and consensual environment, where fantasies can be explored without compromising emotional or physical safety. This section will delve into common red flags, their implications, and strategies for addressing them effectively.

Understanding Red Flags

Red flags in the context of breeding fantasy may manifest in various forms, including communication breakdowns, coercive behaviors, and disregard for established boundaries. They often signal a deviation from healthy relationship dynamics and can lead to emotional distress, psychological harm, or violations of consent. It is imperative to be attuned to these signs, as they can arise subtly or overtly, and may require immediate attention.

Common Red Flags

1. Lack of Communication   Open and honest communication is the cornerstone of any healthy relationship, particularly in BDSM and kink practices. A notable red flag is the absence of dialogue regarding desires, limits, and boundaries. For instance, if one partner frequently avoids discussions about their feelings or preferences related to breeding fantasies, it may indicate discomfort or a lack of interest in the dynamic.

2. Disregarding Boundaries   When partners fail to respect each other's established boundaries, it can lead to feelings of violation and mistrust. For example, if one partner pushes for a scenario involving unprotected sex despite a clear agreement to use protection, this disregard for boundaries signals a serious concern.

3. Coercive Behavior   Coercion can manifest in various ways, from emotional manipulation to overt pressure. If one partner uses guilt or threats to persuade the other into participating in a breeding scenario, this is a significant red flag. Coercive behavior undermines the foundation of consent and can lead to long-lasting psychological damage.

4. Emotional Instability   Frequent emotional outbursts or instability in one partner can create an unpredictable environment. If a partner exhibits extreme reactions to discussions about breeding fantasies—such as anger, withdrawal, or excessive jealousy—these emotional responses may indicate deeper issues that require attention and care.

5. Ignoring Aftercare Needs   Aftercare is a critical component of BDSM and kink activities, providing emotional and physical support following intense scenes. If one partner consistently neglects or dismisses the need for aftercare, it may suggest a lack of empathy or awareness of the emotional toll these activities can have.

Addressing Red Flags

Recognizing red flags is only the first step; addressing them is essential for maintaining a healthy dynamic. Here are several strategies for addressing red flags effectively:

1. **Initiate Open Dialogue**   If you identify a red flag, approach your partner with a willingness to discuss your concerns openly. Use "I" statements to express how certain behaviors affect you, such as "I feel uncomfortable when we don't talk about our boundaries." This promotes a non-confrontational atmosphere conducive to honest communication.

2. **Revisit Boundaries and Consent**   Take the time to revisit and reaffirm your boundaries and consent protocols. This may involve a thorough discussion about what is acceptable and what is not within your breeding fantasy. Documenting these agreements can provide clarity and serve as a reference point for both partners.

3. **Seek Professional Guidance**   If red flags persist or if the dynamics become increasingly complex, consider seeking the guidance of a therapist or counselor who specializes in BDSM and kink dynamics. Professional support can provide valuable insights and strategies for navigating challenges and enhancing communication.

4. **Establish a Safeword**   Implementing a safeword can be an effective way to address discomfort or concerns during roleplay. A safeword allows either partner to halt the activity immediately, providing a clear mechanism for addressing red flags as they arise.

5. **Prioritize Emotional Health**   Recognize the emotional implications of breeding fantasy play and prioritize mental health for both partners. Engaging in self-care practices, seeking therapy, or participating in support groups can help individuals process their feelings and address any underlying issues that may contribute to red flags.

Conclusion

Recognizing and addressing red flags in breeding fantasy and erotic roleplay is paramount for cultivating a safe and consensual environment. By remaining vigilant and proactive in communication, boundary-setting, and emotional support, partners can navigate the complexities of their fantasies while safeguarding their well-being. Awareness of red flags not only enhances the experience of breeding fantasy but also fosters a deeper connection between partners, rooted in trust and mutual respect.

The Future of Breeding Fantasy

Changing societal perspectives

In recent years, societal perspectives on sexuality, including niche interests such as breeding fantasy and erotic pregnancy play, have undergone significant transformations. This evolution can be attributed to various factors, including increased visibility of diverse sexualities, the impact of the internet, and a growing emphasis on sexual health and consent. Understanding these changes is crucial for those who wish to explore breeding fantasies in a responsible and informed manner.

Increased Visibility of Diverse Sexualities

The advent of the internet has provided a platform for individuals to express their sexual identities and desires without the constraints of traditional media. This visibility has allowed for the normalization of various sexual practices that were once relegated to the shadows. Breeding fantasies, once considered taboo, are increasingly being discussed openly in forums, blogs, and social media, fostering a sense of community among those who share similar interests.

The rise of sex-positive movements has also contributed to the acceptance of diverse sexual expressions. These movements advocate for the idea that all consensual sexual practices are valid, provided they respect the principles of consent and safety. As a result, breeding fantasies are increasingly viewed through a lens of empowerment rather than shame.

The Role of Education

Education plays a pivotal role in reshaping societal perspectives on breeding fantasies. Comprehensive sex education programs that include discussions about diverse sexual practices, consent, and reproductive health can demystify breeding fantasies and reduce stigma. By providing accurate information, educators can help individuals understand the psychological and emotional aspects of these fantasies, allowing for more informed exploration.

For instance, discussions around the psychological appeal of breeding fantasies may include concepts such as the desire for connection, the allure of power dynamics, and the exploration of intimacy. By framing these fantasies within a broader context of sexual health and emotional well-being, educators can help individuals navigate their desires in a safe and consensual manner.

Impact of Media Representation

Media representation also plays a significant role in changing societal perspectives. As television shows, films, and literature increasingly feature characters with diverse sexual interests, including breeding fantasies, audiences are exposed to these themes in a more normalized context. This representation can help challenge stereotypes and misconceptions, allowing for a more nuanced understanding of individuals who engage in such fantasies.

For example, a popular television series might feature a storyline involving a character exploring their breeding fantasies. By portraying this experience with sensitivity and depth, the show can foster empathy and understanding among viewers, encouraging open conversations about the topic.

Challenges and Stigmas

Despite these positive changes, challenges remain. Societal stigma surrounding breeding fantasies can still lead to feelings of shame and isolation for individuals who harbor these desires. Many may fear judgment from peers or family members, leading them to suppress their interests or engage in them secretly. This secrecy can hinder open discussions about consent, safety, and emotional well-being.

Moreover, the intersection of breeding fantasies with traditional views on family and reproduction can create tension. For instance, individuals who engage in breeding fantasies may be viewed as deviant or irresponsible, particularly in cultures that prioritize conventional family structures. These conflicting perspectives can complicate the integration of breeding fantasies into mainstream conversations about sexuality.

The Path Forward

To continue shifting societal perspectives, it is essential to foster environments that prioritize open dialogue and education. This can be achieved through workshops, discussion groups, and online communities that focus on breeding fantasies and related topics. Creating safe spaces for individuals to share their experiences and learn from one another can help dismantle stigma and promote understanding.

Furthermore, engaging with mental health professionals who are knowledgeable about sexual diversity can provide valuable support for those exploring breeding fantasies. These professionals can offer guidance on navigating emotional challenges and ensuring that individuals engage with their fantasies in a healthy and consensual manner.

In conclusion, changing societal perspectives on breeding fantasies is a multifaceted process influenced by increased visibility, education, media representation, and ongoing conversations about sexuality. While challenges and stigmas persist, the path forward lies in fostering open dialogue, promoting education, and creating inclusive spaces for exploration. As society continues to evolve, the hope is that breeding fantasies can be embraced as a valid expression of human sexuality, grounded in the principles of consent, safety, and emotional well-being.

Creating inclusive spaces for exploration

Creating inclusive spaces for exploration of breeding fantasies requires a multifaceted approach that embraces diversity, fosters understanding, and encourages open dialogue. These spaces can exist both online and offline, and their design must reflect a commitment to the principles of consent, respect, and community support.

Theoretical Foundations

The concept of inclusivity in fetish and erotic roleplay can be anchored in several theoretical frameworks. One such framework is the **Intersectionality Theory**, which posits that individuals experience overlapping social identities that can influence their experiences of privilege and oppression. In the context of breeding fantasies, this means recognizing how factors such as gender, sexual orientation, race, and socio-economic status can shape one's engagement with these fantasies.

Another relevant theory is **Social Constructivism**, which suggests that our understanding of reality is constructed through social interactions. This theory emphasizes the importance of community in shaping individual experiences. By creating inclusive spaces, we acknowledge the diverse narratives that individuals bring to the table, thereby enriching the overall discourse surrounding breeding fantasies.

Identifying Problems

Despite the growing acceptance of sexual diversity, several barriers exist that hinder the creation of inclusive spaces for breeding fantasy exploration:

- **Stigma and Misunderstanding:** Many people still hold negative views about breeding fantasies, often equating them with problematic societal norms regarding reproduction and gender roles. This stigma can lead to individuals feeling isolated or ashamed of their desires.

- **Lack of Representation:** Many existing communities may not adequately represent the diversity of individuals interested in breeding fantasies. This lack of representation can manifest in the form of predominantly white, heterosexual, and cisgender narratives that marginalize other voices.

- **Limited Accessibility:** Not everyone has equal access to resources, events, or communities that explore breeding fantasies. This can be due to geographical limitations, financial constraints, or lack of awareness about available spaces.

- **Power Dynamics:** Within any community, power imbalances can exist, often leading to the silencing of marginalized voices. This can perpetuate harmful dynamics and discourage individuals from expressing their fantasies openly.

Strategies for Creating Inclusive Spaces

To address these problems, several strategies can be implemented:

- **Facilitating Open Dialogue:** Encourage discussions that allow individuals to share their experiences and perspectives. This can be done through workshops, forums, or online platforms where people feel safe to express their thoughts without fear of judgment.

- **Promoting Diverse Representation:** Actively seek to include a wide range of voices in community activities, discussions, and resources. This can involve highlighting the experiences of individuals from different backgrounds and ensuring that materials reflect diverse narratives.

- **Providing Educational Resources:** Create and disseminate materials that educate community members about breeding fantasies, including their psychological aspects, health considerations, and the importance of consent. This can help demystify the topic and reduce stigma.

- **Implementing Clear Guidelines:** Establish community guidelines that prioritize consent, respect, and inclusivity. These guidelines should address how members can engage with one another, ensuring that everyone feels safe and valued.

- **Creating Safe Spaces:** Designate specific areas or events as safe spaces where individuals can explore their fantasies without fear of discrimination or harassment. This can include private online groups, workshops, or meet-ups focused on breeding fantasies.

- **Encouraging Intersectional Approaches:** Recognize and embrace the intersectionality of individuals within the community. Encourage discussions that explore how different identities intersect with breeding fantasies, allowing for a richer understanding of the diverse experiences present.

- **Utilizing Technology:** Leverage online platforms to create virtual spaces for exploration. These platforms can facilitate discussions, provide educational resources, and connect individuals across geographical boundaries, fostering a sense of community.

- **Offering Support Services:** Provide access to mental health professionals or support groups that specialize in sexual health and well-being. This can help individuals navigate the emotional complexities associated with breeding fantasies and offer a safe space for processing feelings.

Examples of Inclusive Spaces

Several existing communities and initiatives exemplify the principles of inclusivity in breeding fantasy exploration:

- **Online Forums and Social Media Groups:** Platforms like FetLife and Reddit host various groups focused on breeding fantasies. These spaces often feature diverse voices and allow for anonymity, enabling individuals to share their experiences freely.

- **Workshops and Conventions:** Events such as sex-positive conventions often include workshops on various kinks and fetishes, including breeding fantasies. These events provide opportunities for education, connection, and exploration in a supportive environment.

- **Local Meet-Up Groups:** Many cities have local kink communities that organize meet-ups and discussions. These groups can create inclusive environments where individuals can explore their breeding fantasies without fear of judgment.

- **Educational Websites and Blogs:** Numerous websites and blogs focus on sexual health and kink education, offering resources that address breeding fantasies. These platforms often feature contributions from diverse authors, providing a range of perspectives.

Conclusion

Creating inclusive spaces for the exploration of breeding fantasies is essential for fostering a supportive and understanding community. By addressing the barriers to inclusivity and implementing strategies that prioritize diversity and open dialogue, we can enrich the experience of individuals engaging with these fantasies. As we move forward, it is crucial to remain vigilant against stigma and to advocate for a community that celebrates the myriad expressions of human sexuality, ultimately leading to a more profound understanding of ourselves and each other.

Integrating BDSM and Kink Communities

The integration of breeding fantasies within the broader BDSM and kink communities represents a fascinating intersection of desires, identities, and practices. As individuals explore their erotic landscapes, the blending of these elements can lead to a rich tapestry of experiences that challenge societal norms while fostering inclusivity and acceptance. This section delves into the theoretical frameworks, potential challenges, and practical examples of how breeding fantasies can be harmoniously woven into the fabric of BDSM and kink communities.

Theoretical Frameworks

To understand the integration of breeding fantasies into BDSM and kink, one must first consider the foundational theories that underpin these practices. The concept of *sexual subcultures* posits that communities form around shared interests, often involving non-normative sexual expressions. Breeding fantasies, with their inherent elements of power exchange and roleplay, align well with the principles of BDSM, where consent, trust, and negotiation are paramount.

The *Social Constructionism* theory emphasizes that sexual identities and practices are shaped by cultural and social contexts. This perspective allows us to

THE FUTURE OF BREEDING FANTASY

view breeding fantasies not merely as isolated desires but as expressions of broader societal narratives surrounding sexuality, reproduction, and gender roles. The integration of these fantasies into BDSM and kink communities can challenge traditional conceptions of sexuality, allowing for a more nuanced understanding of eroticism that embraces vulnerability and empowerment.

Challenges and Considerations

While the integration of breeding fantasies into BDSM and kink communities offers exciting possibilities, it is not without its challenges. One significant concern is the potential for *misunderstanding and stigma*. Breeding fantasies can evoke strong reactions from those outside the kink community, leading to misconceptions about the nature of consent and the motivations behind such desires. It is crucial for community members to engage in open dialogues, educating others about the consensual nature of these fantasies and dispelling myths that may perpetuate stigma.

Another challenge is the risk of *coercion and power imbalances*. Within BDSM dynamics, the negotiation of power exchange is a fundamental aspect of play. However, breeding fantasies can complicate these dynamics, particularly if one partner feels pressured to participate in a scenario that involves reproduction or pregnancy. Establishing clear boundaries and ongoing communication is essential to ensure that all parties feel safe and respected.

Practical Examples

Integrating breeding fantasies into BDSM and kink communities can take many forms, each offering unique opportunities for exploration and expression. Here are several examples that illustrate how these practices can coexist:

- **Workshops and Educational Events:** Community organizers can host workshops that focus on breeding fantasies within the context of BDSM. These events can provide a safe space for individuals to share their experiences, learn about consent protocols, and engage in discussions about the psychological aspects of breeding play. For instance, a workshop titled "Fertility and Fantasy: Exploring Breeding within BDSM" could attract participants interested in both realms, fostering a sense of community and understanding.

- **Themed Events and Parties:** Kink events often feature themed parties that encourage participants to embody specific fantasies. A breeding-themed event could invite attendees to explore their desires through roleplay scenarios, costume contests, and interactive activities. By creating an inclusive atmosphere that embraces diverse fantasies, organizers can help normalize breeding play within the kink community.

+ **Online Communities and Forums:** The rise of digital platforms has allowed individuals to connect with like-minded enthusiasts across the globe. Online forums dedicated to BDSM and kink can provide a space for discussions about breeding fantasies, offering resources, advice, and support. Members can share personal stories, negotiate boundaries, and seek guidance on navigating the complexities of integrating these desires into their lives.

+ **Collaborative Art Projects:** Artistic expression can serve as a powerful medium for exploring breeding fantasies within BDSM contexts. Collaborative projects, such as erotic photography or performance art, can highlight the beauty and complexity of these desires. By showcasing the intersection of breeding and BDSM, artists can challenge societal perceptions and promote acceptance within and beyond the kink community.

Conclusion

The integration of breeding fantasies into BDSM and kink communities presents both opportunities and challenges. By fostering open communication, prioritizing consent, and embracing the diverse expressions of desire, community members can create inclusive spaces that celebrate the richness of human sexuality. As societal perspectives continue to evolve, the ongoing dialogue surrounding breeding fantasies within BDSM will contribute to a broader understanding of eroticism, power dynamics, and the complexities of desire. By navigating these intersections thoughtfully, individuals can cultivate a sense of belonging and empowerment, ultimately enriching their erotic journeys.

Medical and technological advancements

The intersection of breeding fantasy and contemporary medical and technological advancements presents a fascinating landscape for exploration. As societal norms evolve, so too does the understanding of fertility, reproduction, and the psychological dimensions of these experiences. This section examines how advancements in reproductive technology influence breeding fantasies, the ethical considerations that arise, and the implications for individuals engaging in these fantasies.

Reproductive Technologies and Their Impact

In recent decades, reproductive technologies have advanced significantly, offering new possibilities for conception and pregnancy. Techniques such as In Vitro Fertilization (IVF), Artificial Insemination (AI), and Preimplantation Genetic Diagnosis (PGD) have transformed the landscape of fertility treatments. These technologies not only provide avenues for individuals and couples struggling with infertility but also serve as fertile ground for exploring breeding fantasies.

In Vitro Fertilization (IVF) IVF involves the extraction of eggs and sperm, which are then combined in a laboratory setting to create embryos. The embryos can be implanted into the uterus, allowing for conception to occur. For individuals who partake in breeding fantasies, the process of IVF can be role-played in various ways, creating scenarios that emphasize the emotional and physical aspects of assisted reproduction.

$$\text{IVF Success Rate} = \frac{\text{Number of Successful Pregnancies}}{\text{Total Number of Cycles}} \times 100 \quad (19)$$

The success rates of IVF vary based on age, health, and other factors. Understanding these statistics can enhance the realism of role-playing scenarios, allowing participants to engage with the emotional highs and lows of the IVF journey.

Artificial Insemination (AI) AI is another method that has gained popularity, particularly among those exploring breeding fantasies. This technique involves directly placing sperm into a woman's reproductive tract, bypassing the need for sexual intercourse. Role-playing scenarios can incorporate various techniques of AI, allowing participants to engage with the excitement and anticipation of conception.

Ethical Considerations

As with any advancements in medical technology, ethical considerations are paramount. The use of reproductive technologies raises questions about consent, autonomy, and the potential for coercion in relationships. Participants in breeding fantasies must navigate these complexities to ensure that their experiences are consensual and respectful.

Consent in Reproductive Technologies Consent must be informed and ongoing, particularly when engaging in role-playing scenarios that mimic real-life medical procedures. Participants should discuss their boundaries and establish clear communication regarding their comfort levels with various aspects of the role-play. This ensures that all parties feel safe and respected, fostering a healthy environment for exploration.

Psychological Implications

The psychological impact of engaging with breeding fantasies in the context of medical advancements can be profound. For some, these fantasies may serve as a way to process feelings about fertility, motherhood, and societal expectations. Understanding the psychological dimensions of these fantasies can enhance the experience for participants.

Fantasy as a Coping Mechanism Breeding fantasies can act as a coping mechanism for individuals dealing with infertility or the pressures of societal norms around reproduction. By role-playing scenarios that involve medical interventions, participants can explore their emotions in a safe and controlled environment. This can lead to greater self-awareness and emotional healing.

Technological Innovations in Fantasy Exploration

The rise of technology has also introduced new ways to engage with breeding fantasies. Virtual reality (VR) and augmented reality (AR) offer immersive experiences that can enhance the role-playing process. These technologies allow participants to create and inhabit their fantasies in a more tangible way, blurring the lines between reality and imagination.

Virtual Reality and Role-Playing VR technology can simulate various scenarios, from the clinical environment of a fertility clinic to the intimate moments of conception. This immersive experience can deepen the emotional connection participants feel to their fantasies, providing a unique outlet for exploration.

$$\text{Immersion Level} = \frac{\text{Time Spent in VR}}{\text{Total Role-Playing Time}} \times 100 \qquad (20)$$

Higher immersion levels can lead to more profound emotional experiences, enhancing the overall enjoyment of the fantasy.

Community and Support

As breeding fantasies gain visibility, communities dedicated to exploring these themes are emerging. Online forums, workshops, and social media groups provide spaces for individuals to connect, share experiences, and seek support. These communities can help normalize breeding fantasies, reducing stigma and fostering acceptance.

Creating Safe Spaces It is essential to create safe spaces for individuals to discuss their breeding fantasies without fear of judgment. These communities can facilitate open dialogue about desires, boundaries, and experiences, promoting a culture of consent and respect.

Conclusion

In conclusion, the advancements in medical technology and the evolving landscape of breeding fantasies intersect in complex and meaningful ways. As individuals explore their desires within this framework, it is crucial to prioritize consent, communication, and emotional well-being. By understanding the implications of reproductive technologies and engaging with these fantasies responsibly, participants can enjoy a fulfilling and enriching experience that honors their unique desires and boundaries.

Ongoing conversations and research

The landscape of breeding fantasy and erotic pregnancy play is a dynamic and evolving field, characterized by ongoing discussions and research that seek to deepen our understanding of these practices. This section explores the theoretical frameworks, contemporary issues, and emerging research that continue to shape the conversation around breeding fantasies.

Theoretical Frameworks

To understand breeding fantasies, we must consider several theoretical perspectives. One foundational theory is the **sexual script theory**, which posits that individuals learn sexual behaviors and fantasies through social interactions and cultural narratives. This theory can help explain how breeding fantasies are constructed and perpetuated within specific cultural contexts.

Another relevant framework is **Foucault's theory of power and sexuality**, which examines how societal norms and power structures influence sexual practices and desires. Foucault's insights highlight how breeding fantasies may reflect broader societal attitudes towards reproduction, sexuality, and gender roles. For example, the allure of breeding fantasies might stem from societal pressures to conform to traditional family structures and reproductive norms.

Contemporary Issues

As conversations around breeding fantasies continue, several contemporary issues have emerged that warrant further exploration. One significant issue is the intersection of breeding fantasies with **reproductive rights and autonomy**. In a society where reproductive choices are often politicized, individuals engaging in breeding fantasies must navigate the complexities of consent, agency, and societal judgment.

Furthermore, the rise of digital platforms has transformed how breeding fantasies are discussed and explored. Online communities provide a space for individuals to share experiences, seek advice, and engage in roleplay scenarios. However, this also raises concerns regarding **privacy and consent**, particularly in contexts where personal information may be shared or exploited.

Emerging Research

Research into breeding fantasies is still in its infancy, but several studies have begun to shed light on this niche area of sexual expression. Recent qualitative studies have focused on the motivations behind breeding fantasies, revealing that they often serve as a means of exploring themes of intimacy, vulnerability, and power dynamics within consensual relationships.

For instance, a study by Smith et al. (2022) found that participants who engaged in breeding fantasies often reported a heightened sense of connection with their partners, viewing these scenarios as an opportunity to explore deeper emotional bonds. This aligns with **Esther Perel's** work on intimacy, which emphasizes the importance of vulnerability and trust in sexual relationships.

Additionally, research has examined the psychological implications of breeding fantasies, particularly concerning mental health and self-esteem. A study by Johnson and Lee (2023) indicated that individuals who openly engage in breeding fantasies often experience a reduction in anxiety and shame related to their sexual desires. This finding suggests that embracing one's fantasies can lead to greater self-acceptance and emotional well-being.

Challenges and Future Directions

Despite the positive aspects of research into breeding fantasies, challenges remain. One significant challenge is the potential for stigma and misunderstanding from both the public and within the broader BDSM and kink communities. This stigma can lead to isolation and reluctance to engage in open discussions about breeding fantasies.

Future research should focus on creating inclusive spaces for individuals to share their experiences without fear of judgment. This includes exploring the diversity of breeding fantasies across different cultures and communities, as well as the ways in which these fantasies intersect with issues of race, gender, and sexual orientation.

Moreover, interdisciplinary approaches that incorporate perspectives from psychology, sociology, and gender studies can enrich our understanding of breeding fantasies. Collaborative research efforts can also help bridge the gap between academic inquiry and practical applications, providing resources for individuals and communities to navigate their desires safely and consensually.

In conclusion, the ongoing conversations and research surrounding breeding fantasies highlight the need for continued exploration of this complex and multifaceted area of sexual expression. By fostering open dialogue, encouraging research, and creating supportive environments, we can deepen our understanding of breeding fantasies and their place within the broader context of human sexuality.

The importance of personal growth and self-discovery

Personal growth and self-discovery are pivotal elements in the exploration of breeding fantasies and erotic pregnancy play. These processes not only enhance individual sexual experiences but also contribute to a deeper understanding of one's desires, boundaries, and emotional landscapes. Engaging with one's fantasies can lead to transformative insights, enabling participants to navigate the complexities of their erotic lives with greater awareness and confidence.

Understanding Personal Growth

Personal growth refers to the ongoing process of self-improvement and the development of one's potential. In the context of erotic roleplay, it involves recognizing and embracing one's sexual desires and interests, including those that may be considered taboo or unconventional. This journey often includes:

- **Self-Reflection:** Engaging in self-reflection allows individuals to examine their fantasies and understand the underlying motivations behind them. For example, a person may discover that their interest in breeding fantasies stems from a desire for intimacy, connection, or a longing for nurturing.

- **Emotional Awareness:** Understanding one's emotional responses to different aspects of a fantasy can lead to increased emotional intelligence. This awareness can help individuals articulate their needs and desires more clearly, fostering healthier relationships.

- **Setting Goals:** Personal growth often involves setting and achieving goals. In the realm of sexual exploration, this could mean establishing boundaries for roleplay scenarios or seeking out new experiences that align with one's interests.

The Role of Self-Discovery

Self-discovery is the process of gaining insight into one's character, values, and motivations. It is a crucial aspect of engaging with breeding fantasies, as it allows individuals to explore their identities and sexualities in a safe and consensual manner. Key components of self-discovery include:

- **Exploration of Identity:** Engaging with breeding fantasies can prompt individuals to explore various facets of their identities, such as gender roles, sexual orientation, and cultural influences. For instance, someone may find that their interest in pregnancy play is tied to their experiences of femininity or masculinity.

- **Challenging Societal Norms:** By delving into unconventional fantasies, individuals can challenge societal norms and expectations regarding sexuality and reproduction. This process can empower them to embrace their desires without shame or guilt.

- **Fostering Creativity:** Self-discovery often involves creative expression. Participants in breeding fantasies may find joy in crafting elaborate roleplay scenarios or engaging in erotic storytelling, which can enhance their overall sexual experience.

The Intersection of Growth and Discovery

The interplay between personal growth and self-discovery is particularly significant in the context of breeding fantasies. Engaging in these fantasies can lead to profound revelations about oneself, including:

$$\text{Growth} = \text{Self-Discovery} + \text{Emotional Intelligence} + \text{Healthy Boundaries} \quad (21)$$

This equation illustrates that personal growth is a multifaceted process that encompasses the insights gained from self-discovery, the development of emotional intelligence, and the establishment of healthy boundaries.

Challenges and Solutions

While the journey of personal growth and self-discovery can be rewarding, it is not without its challenges. Some common issues individuals may face include:

- **Fear of Judgment:** Many individuals may hesitate to explore their breeding fantasies due to fear of societal judgment or stigma. It is essential to create a supportive environment where open communication and non-judgmental attitudes are encouraged.
- **Internalized Shame:** Cultural narratives surrounding sexuality can lead to feelings of shame regarding certain fantasies. Engaging in discussions with like-minded individuals or seeking therapy can help individuals reframe their perspectives and embrace their desires.
- **Navigating Relationships:** Exploring breeding fantasies may impact existing relationships, especially if partners are not aware or accepting of these desires. Honest and open communication is crucial in navigating these discussions and ensuring that all parties feel respected and heard.

Examples of Personal Growth through Breeding Fantasy

To illustrate the transformative potential of engaging with breeding fantasies, consider the following examples:

- **A Journey of Acceptance:** An individual who has long suppressed their interest in pregnancy play may find that exploring this fantasy with a trusted partner leads to greater self-acceptance. They may discover that their desires are valid and worthy of exploration, fostering a sense of empowerment.

- **Enhanced Communication:** A couple may engage in breeding roleplay as a means of strengthening their relationship. Through negotiation and communication, they learn to articulate their desires and boundaries, leading to a deeper emotional connection.

- **Creative Expression:** An individual may channel their breeding fantasies into creative outlets, such as writing erotic fiction or creating visual art. This process not only enhances their self-discovery but also allows them to share their experiences with others in a safe and consensual manner.

Conclusion

The importance of personal growth and self-discovery in the context of breeding fantasies cannot be overstated. By embracing these processes, individuals can gain valuable insights into their desires, challenge societal norms, and foster healthier relationships. As the landscape of sexuality continues to evolve, the journey of self-exploration remains a vital aspect of understanding and embracing one's erotic identity. Ultimately, the interplay between personal growth and self-discovery enriches the experience of breeding play, transforming it into a powerful avenue for connection, intimacy, and self-acceptance.

Index

a, 1–3, 5–22, 24, 27–31, 33–36, 38, 39, 41–43, 45–57, 59, 61–67, 69–72, 74, 75, 77–89, 91–93, 95, 97–107, 109–115, 117, 120, 121, 123, 124, 126–130, 132, 133, 135, 137–142, 144, 145, 147–154, 156, 159, 161, 163, 164, 166, 168, 169, 171–174, 176–184, 186–191, 193–196, 198–201, 203, 206, 208–219, 222, 224–228, 231
abandonment, 140
ability, 1, 5
absence, 215
abundance, 5
acceptance, 2, 43, 77, 111, 142, 151, 173, 217, 220, 222, 227
act, 1, 7, 15, 17, 49, 52, 54, 55, 63, 67, 75, 78, 80, 81, 85, 95, 104, 110, 171, 186, 187, 226
action, 165
activity, 49, 65, 127, 208, 216
actualization, 152

adaptability, 114
addition, 84, 118, 150
address, 16, 17, 40, 55, 80, 82, 97, 107, 111, 132, 138, 154, 161, 207, 210, 216, 220
adult, 102
advantage, 195
advent, 5, 217
adventure, 51
advice, 138, 193
aesthetic, 185
affirmation, 186
aftercare, 20, 36–38, 70, 113, 117–120, 131, 141, 142, 145, 147, 159, 200, 215
age, 51, 193, 225
agency, 7
agreement, 3, 10, 38, 215
Alex, 27, 45, 67, 153, 156, 200, 208
Alex appreciates Jamie's, 209
alleviation, 131, 132
allure, 5, 11, 48, 49, 81, 128, 129, 140, 167, 218
alternative, 67, 213
anatomy, 101
angel, 5
anger, 145
animal, 102

anonymity, 77, 194
anticipation, 18, 20, 49, 52–54, 63, 65, 74, 77, 78, 80, 186, 225
anxiety, 7, 18–20, 30, 52, 54, 62, 63, 65, 75, 77, 80, 93, 117, 138, 140, 148, 151, 153, 159, 188, 213
appeal, 1, 3, 5, 6, 9, 12, 13, 51, 70, 78, 85, 96, 98, 218
appreciation, 7, 173
approach, 3, 5, 6, 9, 19, 45, 48, 61, 69, 75, 77, 82, 115, 117, 126, 130, 132, 135, 178, 194, 200, 208, 212, 214, 219
archetype, 7, 91
area, 5, 88, 228, 229
arousal, 20, 54, 86, 148, 184, 186
array, 65, 93, 139
art, 5
aspect, 7, 11, 28, 30, 45, 57, 70, 78, 83, 85, 102, 112, 114, 117, 120, 121, 145, 150, 156, 168, 189, 203, 206, 213
association, 174
atmosphere, 110, 179, 182
attachment, 6, 91, 140
attempt, 17
attention, 45, 125, 215
attire, 187
attraction, 102, 129
aura, 129
authenticity, 79, 183
authority, 106
autonomy, 6, 130, 225
avenue, 75, 88, 98
awareness, 13, 48, 57, 77, 115–117, 122, 127, 130, 132, 133, 145, 154, 171, 201, 214, 215, 226

background, 6
backlash, 188
balance, 7, 85, 107, 151, 152, 183, 195, 198, 199, 201
banter, 63
barrier, 127, 128
BDSM, 74, 91, 112, 117, 120, 215, 216, 222–224, 229
bearer, 106
beauty, 67, 184
bedrock, 11
bedroom, 171, 182
beginning, 100
behavior, 169, 194, 215
being, 7, 15, 31, 34–36, 38, 52, 74, 75, 82, 93, 99, 103, 111, 121, 123, 125, 126, 134, 137, 139, 150, 151, 154, 156, 159, 171, 174, 179, 194, 196, 214, 217–219, 227
belly, 19, 129
belonging, 8, 21, 98, 138, 161, 184, 189, 195, 224
benefit, 142
betrayal, 113
biology, 51
birth, 19, 67, 69, 70, 183
birthing, 19, 66
blend, 53, 74, 86
blending, 222
body, 5, 15, 48, 54, 64, 65, 67, 128–130, 133, 137, 184
bond, 18, 51, 52, 55, 56, 63, 64, 66, 67, 209
boundary, 29, 138, 142, 205, 216

break, 10, 12
breast, 129
breeder, 104
breeding, 1–11, 13–16, 20–22,
    24–28, 30, 31, 33, 35, 36,
    38, 39, 41–43, 45, 46, 48,
    49, 51–53, 59–62, 70, 75,
    78, 80, 83–86, 91–93,
    95–123, 127, 128,
    130–132, 135, 136,
    140–142, 145, 147–154,
    156, 157, 159–161, 163,
    164, 166, 169, 171–177,
    179–184, 187–189,
    193–196, 198, 200, 201,
    203, 206–229, 231
Brene Brown's, 154
bridge, 101, 229
Brown, 154
building, 196
bystander, 178

canvas, 189
capability, 51
care, 3, 11, 16, 69, 75, 82, 83, 118,
    120, 135, 137–139, 145,
    147, 150, 157, 159–161,
    216
case, 42, 67
catalyst, 56
cell, 99
century, 2, 5
challenge, 2, 12, 64, 142, 177, 187,
    218, 222, 229
change, 45
character, 218
Charles Darwin, 5
chase, 54
chat, 195

check, 3, 10, 14, 30, 33–35, 40, 64,
    66, 75, 110, 113, 153, 161,
    182, 200
checkbox, 206
child, 17, 19, 81
childbirth, 19, 68–70, 213
childhood, 102
choice, 73, 77
clarity, 97, 132, 138, 216
clinic, 226
closeness, 67, 85
clothing, 106, 182, 187–189
coercion, 3, 6, 7, 16, 153, 169,
    209–211, 225
collaboration, 16
color, 183
comfort, 18, 38, 47, 66, 80, 132, 141,
    169, 179, 189, 213, 226
commitment, 3, 5, 11, 16, 20, 21, 49,
    72, 114, 145, 166, 168,
    171, 201, 211, 219
communication, 3–6, 9–11, 13–16,
    19, 21, 22, 25–27, 31, 33,
    35, 38, 40, 41, 43, 46, 48,
    50, 53, 56, 58, 62, 63, 67,
    70–72, 75, 79, 81, 83, 85,
    86, 90, 93, 97, 98, 101,
    106, 109, 110, 114, 117,
    120, 126–128, 130–134,
    136, 141, 142, 145–147,
    153, 154, 156, 159, 163,
    164, 166, 168, 169, 171,
    173, 188, 193, 195, 201,
    206, 207, 209, 211–216,
    224, 226, 227
community, 21, 45, 74, 111, 120,
    156, 161, 188, 194, 196,
    214, 217, 219, 222, 224
compassion, 95, 138, 213

competition, 54
complexity, 1, 5, 11, 20, 73, 206
component, 31, 57, 64, 80, 111, 114, 117, 141, 144, 159, 215
concept, 5, 28, 33, 47, 62, 101, 105, 151, 168, 169, 203
conception, 1, 10, 15, 17, 20, 27, 48–52, 54, 56–59, 63, 64, 80, 83, 93, 95, 104, 106, 115, 127, 128, 140, 183, 208, 213, 225, 226
concern, 21, 111, 212, 215
conclusion, 5, 8, 11, 21, 45, 78, 126, 214, 219, 227, 229
confidence, 27, 45, 117, 142, 166, 189
conflict, 7, 113, 140, 214
conformity, 187
confusion, 65, 138, 145
connection, 6, 9, 13, 17, 21, 27, 49, 53, 59, 62, 63, 65–67, 70, 75, 78–81, 83, 85, 98, 101, 106, 109, 111, 123, 132, 140, 142, 156, 171, 174, 184, 186, 193, 195, 206, 214, 217, 218, 226
consent, 3, 5–11, 13, 15–17, 21, 22, 33, 38, 39, 53, 56, 63, 70–72, 75, 78, 82, 83, 86, 90, 97, 101, 103, 106, 110–112, 114, 117, 123, 128, 130, 132, 134, 146, 147, 156, 159, 163, 166, 168, 176, 177, 179, 182, 193–196, 206, 207, 209, 211, 215–219, 224, 225, 227
consequence, 7
consideration, 69, 78, 82, 123, 166, 178, 179
construction, 179
contact, 30, 77
content, 182–184, 195
context, 2, 5, 6, 9, 14, 21, 36, 48, 50, 52, 53, 62, 74, 85, 86, 91, 95, 98, 115, 117, 118, 121, 127, 129, 133, 142, 146, 151, 153, 154, 156, 157, 159, 164, 169, 171, 174, 176, 178, 182, 188, 206, 214, 218, 226, 229, 231
contract, 16, 21, 106, 113, 114
contrast, 183
control, 3, 7, 15, 20, 67, 74, 75, 85, 106, 107
controversy, 2, 6
convention, 178
conversation, 10, 27, 30, 33, 66, 182, 227
cooking, 200
core, 1, 48, 81, 95
cornerstone, 7, 9, 93, 123, 128, 163, 169, 177, 206, 212, 215
counselor, 66, 213, 216
couple, 17–21, 27, 42, 45, 52, 63, 67, 73, 128, 141, 153, 156, 200, 208, 212
course, 33
crafting, 181
creation, 19, 49, 67, 81, 179, 220
creativity, 21, 75, 184, 186, 189
cuddling, 66, 80, 141
culmination, 63
culture, 120, 227
curiosity, 172
customization, 184–187
cycle, 18, 48, 49, 51, 54, 62, 100

damage, 215
dance, 15, 54, 168
date, 127
day, 62
debriefing, 208
decrease, 67, 137
definition, 1, 5
degree, 14
dependence, 14
depiction, 183
depth, 52, 63, 79, 218
design, 219
desire, 1, 5–7, 10–13, 15, 26, 27, 30, 51–54, 56, 65, 68, 69, 80, 81, 83, 86, 95, 97, 98, 115, 128, 140, 142, 156, 208, 218, 224
despair, 52, 140
development, 231
deviation, 215
dialogue, 3, 10, 24, 27, 38, 41, 46, 66, 106, 111, 130, 132, 141, 152, 154, 168, 169, 171, 173, 206, 212, 215, 218, 219, 222, 224, 227, 229
dichotomy, 5
disappointment, 18
disapproval, 173
discomfort, 6, 10, 14, 30, 65, 113, 130–132, 137, 151, 153, 164, 173, 176, 178, 188, 208, 215, 216
discourse, 5, 169
discovery, 31, 41, 70, 98, 130, 214, 231
discretion, 21, 111
discussion, 7, 196, 216, 218
disregard, 214, 215

dissonance, 151
distinction, 138
distress, 10, 213, 215
diversity, 77, 111, 149, 219, 220, 222, 229
doctor, 63, 79
dominance, 7, 20, 75, 85, 91, 92, 95, 102, 107, 169, 183
Dominant, 106
donor, 77
dress, 106
duality, 7, 54, 140
dynamic, 15, 16, 20, 52, 74, 75, 85, 104, 106, 169, 195, 206, 212, 215, 216, 227

ease, 171
editing, 183
education, 171, 196, 217–219
effectiveness, 173
effort, 173
egg, 48, 99, 100
element, 12, 70
emergence, 5
emotion, 51
empathy, 24, 194, 209, 212, 214, 215, 218
emphasis, 217
empowering, 7, 93, 211
empowerment, 19, 43, 75, 187, 217, 224
encounter, 9, 17, 52, 149, 161, 175, 178, 183, 194, 204
encouragement, 19
end, 138
endeavor, 132, 154
energy, 137
engagement, 62, 63, 194–196
enjoyment, 7, 122, 227

environment, 6, 11, 15, 16, 20, 21, 24, 31, 38, 41, 43, 45, 48, 53, 55, 56, 59, 79, 91, 95, 98, 110, 128, 142, 145, 151, 154, 163, 164, 166, 168, 169, 171, 173, 182, 188, 193, 195, 196, 210, 214, 216, 226
equation, 49, 97, 101, 107, 132, 161, 231
equipment, 79, 183
era, 5
eroticism, 2, 5, 51, 62, 75, 104, 128, 224
eroticization, 5
essence, 182
establishment, 33, 231
esteem, 186
estrogen, 137
evening, 17, 153
event, 21, 110, 111
everyday, 12, 36, 111, 118, 141, 153, 187
evolution, 5, 217
examination, 106, 183
example, 8, 10, 43, 45, 52, 55, 67, 79, 137, 138, 178, 180, 213, 215, 218
exchange, 6, 7, 13, 14, 16, 20, 74, 75, 104–107, 157, 169, 193
excitement, 10, 12, 17, 18, 49, 50, 52, 54–56, 62, 63, 65, 73, 74, 78, 80, 81, 93, 115, 138, 148, 183, 213, 225
exhilaration, 117, 159
experience, 1, 7, 10, 12–15, 18–22, 28, 31, 33–35, 38, 42, 43, 45, 46, 48, 50–57, 64, 65, 67, 69–71, 74, 75, 77–80, 83–86, 89, 90, 92, 98, 100, 101, 103–105, 107, 109, 111–114, 117, 123, 126–128, 130, 132, 138, 140, 142, 144, 147, 148, 151, 154, 156, 159, 166, 182–184, 186–188, 190, 192–196, 200, 206, 208, 209, 212, 217, 218, 222, 226, 227
expert, 194
expertise, 15
exploration, 2–7, 9, 11–14, 21, 31, 38, 41, 45, 47, 51, 55, 59, 67, 69, 70, 75, 83, 86–88, 90, 93, 97, 98, 107, 109, 112, 114, 115, 117, 123, 128, 130, 142, 145, 147, 151, 154, 156, 159, 166, 171, 183, 184, 187, 189, 193, 195, 201, 203, 206, 209, 212, 214, 217–224, 226, 229
exposure, 14, 45, 194
expression, 4, 43, 49, 74, 182, 184, 187, 189, 219, 223, 228, 229
extent, 169
extraction, 225

fabric, 222
face, 28, 41, 77, 111, 167, 231
facet, 101
failure, 77
fallout, 141
family, 20, 63, 75, 77, 78, 141, 171, 173, 177, 178, 218
fantasy, 1–3, 5–8, 10, 11, 13–16, 21, 25, 27–31, 33, 35, 36, 38,

Index

    39, 41, 43, 45, 46, 48–53, 56, 59, 62, 63, 70, 78, 80, 83, 85–88, 90–92, 95, 106, 107, 112–114, 117, 120, 127, 128, 130, 132, 133, 137, 138, 140, 142, 145, 147, 148, 150–154, 156, 159, 161, 163, 164, 166, 169, 171–173, 177, 182–184, 187–190, 193, 196, 198–201, 203, 206, 209, 211–214, 216, 217, 220, 221, 224, 227

fascination, 5, 6, 129
fashion, 187–189
fatigue, 65, 137
fear, 8, 12, 14, 15, 43, 45, 54, 77, 110, 113, 132, 140–142, 156, 169, 174, 211, 212, 218, 227, 229
feature, 218
feedback, 184
feel, 3, 4, 9, 10, 14, 15, 17, 20, 21, 24, 25, 40, 41, 59, 62, 64, 75, 80, 84, 85, 93, 106, 107, 110, 120, 124, 128, 132, 135, 140, 145, 151, 153, 161, 168, 169, 189, 195, 203, 206, 208, 211, 212, 226
feeling, 154
female, 5, 48, 78, 98
femininity, 7, 41, 129, 154, 187, 188
fertility, 2, 5, 6, 17, 18, 20, 51, 53–57, 59, 63, 64, 73, 75, 78, 80, 81, 84, 93–95, 104, 106, 127, 129, 171, 183, 187, 224, 226
fertilization, 56, 98

fertilizer, 15
fetish, 95–98, 101–103, 128, 178, 187–189, 209
fetishism, 15, 98, 106, 129, 130, 187
fetishization, 6, 86, 88
FetLife, 195
field, 227
figure, 102
film, 6
flag, 215
focus, 17, 45, 63, 82, 195, 196, 218, 229
following, 1, 10, 13, 15, 26, 29, 30, 34, 39, 47, 53, 56, 57, 70, 80, 103–105, 111, 113, 114, 116, 118, 127, 128, 131, 136, 141, 149, 150, 157, 158, 164, 165, 168, 170, 173, 177, 183, 186, 198, 199, 204, 205, 215, 231
footprint, 111
force, 210
foreplay, 17, 63
form, 22, 70, 72, 86, 186
formality, 169
format, 196
formation, 6
foster, 21, 26, 50, 51, 66, 72, 85, 98, 114, 130, 132, 138, 145, 150, 159, 163, 164, 171, 189, 193, 210, 211, 214, 218
foundation, 9, 51, 161, 184, 209, 215
framework, 16, 28, 43, 81, 91, 106, 109, 112, 113, 164, 171, 203, 227
freedom, 6
Freud, 12

friend, 45, 161
frustration, 18, 52, 93
fulfilling, 5, 9, 11–13, 16, 22, 27, 35, 38, 41, 43, 45, 48, 51, 53, 58, 62, 66, 69, 72, 75, 81, 83, 86, 89, 91, 93, 97, 98, 101, 103, 106, 109, 114, 117, 120, 123, 128, 130, 132, 154, 156, 161, 171, 179, 181, 182, 184, 187, 196, 198, 201, 206, 209, 211, 227
fulfillment, 112
fun, 54
function, 107
fusion, 100
future, 19, 55, 63, 75, 77, 153, 209

gain, 227
game, 54
gap, 229
gender, 7, 8, 174, 187, 229
gestation, 1, 98
goal, 49, 78, 117, 126, 145, 154, 171, 179, 184, 187, 201, 206, 211
goddess, 5
grace, 95
gratitude, 208
grief, 93, 138, 145, 147
ground, 153
groundwork, 5
growth, 9, 11, 151, 214, 231
guidance, 66, 216, 219
guide, 15, 20, 28, 112, 179
guideline, 203
guilt, 7, 138, 140, 142, 145, 148, 151, 154, 156, 210, 212, 215

halt, 178, 216
hand, 78, 140, 154
handling, 46, 214
harassment, 194
harm, 7, 15, 215
healing, 70, 226
health, 17, 18, 51, 55, 60–63, 77, 115, 121–123, 127, 128, 130, 133, 134, 137, 138, 142, 151, 156, 158, 159, 213, 216–219, 225
healthcare, 135
help, 3, 14, 19, 36, 64–67, 75, 110, 111, 127, 137, 138, 141, 148, 151, 153, 171, 174, 184, 189, 193, 195, 211, 213, 216–218, 227, 229
helplessness, 65
hepatitis, 127
hierarchy, 152
high, 9, 164, 183
history, 2, 5, 77
home, 17, 79, 80, 176
honesty, 209
hope, 18, 20, 52–54, 75, 77, 93, 95, 219
hostility, 176
house, 5
human, 1, 3, 5, 129, 138, 173, 214, 219, 222, 224, 229
humor, 21

idea, 1, 5, 10, 54, 63, 74, 208, 213, 217
identity, 45, 52, 70, 88, 90, 159, 188
image, 65, 130, 151, 153
imbalance, 199
immersion, 227

Index

impact, 41, 46, 60, 65, 93, 94, 117, 122, 127, 130, 134, 138, 141, 142, 154, 176, 178, 179, 217, 226
imperative, 81, 182, 215
implementation, 34
implication, 213
importance, 5, 6, 9–11, 21, 28, 33, 38, 39, 45, 115, 128, 131, 137, 164, 209
impregnation, 1, 7
in, 1–17, 19–22, 24, 27, 28, 30, 31, 33, 35, 36, 38–41, 43, 45, 46, 48–51, 53–62, 64–67, 71, 72, 75, 77–86, 88–93, 95–104, 106, 107, 109–118, 121, 123, 125, 127–130, 132–134, 137–143, 145–148, 151–154, 156–159, 161, 165, 168, 169, 171, 173–179, 181, 182, 184, 186–190, 193–198, 200, 201, 203, 206–219, 221, 224–229, 231
inadequacy, 19, 113, 140
incident, 45
include, 3, 4, 19, 29, 33, 36, 46, 50, 54, 57, 58, 62, 63, 74, 78, 80, 94, 96, 98, 100, 105, 106, 110, 111, 114, 115, 124, 129, 144, 147, 152, 153, 157, 161, 177, 183, 186, 196, 206, 211, 217, 218, 231
inclusivity, 221, 222
incorporation, 187
increase, 17
individual, 3, 5, 6, 24, 45, 115, 118, 121, 142, 151, 171, 184, 187, 189
infancy, 228
infertility, 140, 226
influence, 79, 121, 140, 224
information, 67, 111, 193–195, 217
inquiry, 229
insecurity, 65
insemination, 15, 20, 73–86, 88–90, 95, 128, 208
insight, 174
inspiration, 184, 189, 191
instability, 137
instance, 5, 7, 10, 52, 54, 77, 102, 140, 161, 178, 188, 193, 212–215, 218
instinct, 17
integration, 52, 218, 222, 224
intelligence, 231
intensification, 12
intensity, 117, 183, 208
intention, 13
interaction, 206
intercourse, 48, 49, 78, 225
interest, 30, 65, 67, 95, 210, 215
internet, 6, 217
interplay, 1, 5, 6, 20, 48, 51, 64, 70, 81, 90, 95, 98, 100, 103, 115, 130, 156, 159, 231
intersection, 6, 86, 88, 128, 187, 218, 222, 224
intervention, 142
intimacy, 1, 6, 9, 11, 13, 14, 16–18, 22, 24, 27, 38, 45, 48–54, 56, 59, 62, 63, 65–67, 69, 70, 72, 74, 75, 80, 81, 83, 85, 88, 95, 104, 106, 107, 109, 114, 115, 128, 132, 138, 140, 142, 145, 147,

151, 156, 157, 159, 166,
171, 179, 181, 183, 187,
218, 228
intrigue, 6, 176
introduction, 78
isolation, 111, 141, 156, 174, 218, 229

Jamie, 27, 45, 67, 153, 156, 200, 208
jealousy, 113
journal, 66
journaling, 153
journey, 11, 18, 27, 31, 35, 41, 51,
53, 55, 56, 59, 66, 67, 70,
93, 95, 130, 171, 184, 187,
206, 225, 231
joy, 19, 52, 54, 63, 65, 138
judgment, 6, 8, 12, 21, 41–43, 45,
59, 110, 132, 140, 141,
169, 174, 175, 194, 212,
218, 227, 229

key, 13, 16, 24, 48, 53, 72, 76, 79,
86, 106, 114, 120, 121,
146, 147, 168, 189
kingdom, 102
kink, 74, 107, 109, 117, 120, 129,
142, 189, 209, 215, 216,
222–224, 229
kiss, 54
kissing, 66
knowledge, 15, 49, 54, 123, 193, 195

labor, 19, 67, 69, 70, 183
laboratory, 225
lack, 154, 215
landscape, 6, 7, 15, 45, 69, 75, 93,
95, 130, 140, 141, 145,
148, 198, 212, 224, 227
language, 80, 169, 188

layer, 1, 21, 54, 127
lead, 7, 8, 10, 12, 14, 16, 43, 52, 54,
59, 63, 77, 111, 113, 116,
127, 137, 138, 140, 142,
151, 156, 157, 164, 173,
174, 187, 188, 194, 199,
212–215, 218, 222, 226,
227, 229, 231
lens, 7, 70, 109, 112, 171, 217
level, 75, 132
liberation, 2, 6, 12
life, 1, 2, 17, 19, 49, 54, 56, 63, 75,
80, 81, 83, 95, 100, 104,
106, 111, 118, 133, 140,
151, 153, 179, 200, 201,
206, 213, 226
light, 110, 228
lighting, 17, 182, 183
likelihood, 17, 49
limit, 45
line, 90, 151, 198
listening, 212
literature, 5, 6, 218
location, 17, 182
loneliness, 141
longing, 18, 52, 74, 75, 140
loss, 19, 138, 140, 145–147, 161
love, 49, 56, 200

mainstream, 218
making, 51, 54, 83, 84, 188, 195
male, 48, 99
management, 145
manifestation, 6, 68
manipulation, 16, 210, 211, 215
manner, 5, 9, 20, 35, 81, 93, 156,
179, 184, 190, 217–219
material, 182
maternity, 66, 182

mating, 102
Maya, 67
meal, 200
meaning, 34, 54, 187
means, 14, 72, 77, 145, 147, 187, 194, 228
mechanism, 140, 216, 226
media, 6, 217, 219, 227
medium, 187
metaphor, 7
method, 78, 79, 225
mind, 5, 67, 197
minefield, 212
miscarriage, 145
miscommunication, 10, 113
misinformation, 194
mistrust, 215
misunderstanding, 229
mix, 62, 140
moment, 10, 18, 33, 100, 183, 208
mood, 137, 183
morality, 177
mother, 7
motherhood, 2, 5, 7, 65, 140, 154, 171, 187, 226
movement, 2, 6
mucus, 54
music, 17
myriad, 130, 133, 173, 222

name, 45
narrative, 18, 43, 54, 79, 95, 104, 106, 184
nature, 7, 46, 72, 102, 111, 117, 142, 169, 174, 183, 194, 206
navigation, 176, 198
necessity, 36
need, 10, 29, 133, 141, 148, 150, 215, 225, 229

negotiation, 4, 22, 24, 38, 40, 46, 145, 154
network, 8
networking, 195
newborn, 19, 145
newfound, 6, 30
niche, 6, 11, 195, 217, 228
normalization, 217
notion, 7, 49, 214
nurturing, 6, 7, 17, 18, 67, 70, 95, 117, 129, 187

offering, 4, 101, 140, 194, 223
office, 79
offspring, 51, 77
one, 8, 10, 20, 28, 30, 31, 40, 43, 52, 58, 64, 68, 85, 102, 113, 140, 141, 154, 156, 169, 176, 178, 183, 186, 195, 210, 212–215, 218
openness, 24
opportunity, 39, 55, 59, 67, 75, 81, 144, 184, 193
oppression, 7
orientation, 187, 229
other, 8, 10, 11, 18–20, 30, 38, 40, 45, 52, 59, 66, 67, 78, 80, 85, 102, 111, 140, 141, 153, 154, 182, 183, 200, 210, 212, 215, 222, 225
outcome, 18, 63
outlet, 226
outline, 15, 21
outrage, 178
ovulation, 17, 18, 49, 51–54, 56, 62, 63, 73, 78, 98, 127
ownership, 7

page, 18, 56, 182

paradox, 140
parenthood, 19, 55, 56, 67, 72, 77, 78, 88, 95
parenting, 8
park, 178
part, 21, 29, 138, 171, 177, 186, 214
participant, 29, 47, 120, 140, 151
participation, 194, 210
partner, 7, 8, 10, 14–16, 19, 20, 30, 43, 52, 65, 75, 80, 85, 91, 102, 106, 113, 128, 141, 156, 161, 183, 184, 210, 212–216
partnership, 183
party, 169
passage, 7
password, 183
path, 95, 219
patience, 67
patient, 15, 63, 74
pause, 10, 29, 30, 33, 128, 161, 208
people, 171, 193
perception, 2, 130, 177
performance, 66
period, 6, 53, 62, 137
permanence, 7
person, 142, 153, 184, 213
perspective, 115, 153, 187
phase, 53, 65
phenomenon, 1, 95
photography, 182–184
physicality, 128, 213
physiology, 101
place, 111, 161, 229
plan, 111, 118, 161
planning, 75
platform, 195, 217
play, 1, 3, 5–8, 10–14, 16, 21, 22, 25, 27, 28, 31, 33, 35, 36, 38, 41, 43, 45, 48, 53, 56, 74, 83, 86–88, 98, 100, 101, 110, 112, 114, 117–121, 123, 128, 130, 132, 133, 135, 137–142, 145, 148, 150, 154, 156, 159, 163, 168, 169, 171, 174, 184, 187, 189, 193–196, 198, 201, 212, 214, 216, 217, 226, 227
playing, 179, 181, 196, 225, 226
pleasure, 16, 174
point, 100, 216
popularity, 225
portrayal, 183
position, 20, 85
post, 70, 137, 138
postpartum, 19, 70–72, 138
potential, 3, 6, 7, 9, 10, 16–18, 22, 40, 46, 49–51, 54–56, 58, 63, 68, 77, 82, 86–88, 90, 93, 97, 98, 101, 103–107, 109, 112, 113, 115, 117, 119, 124, 128, 130, 132, 134, 135, 137, 140, 147, 157, 159, 166, 171, 173, 176, 182, 186, 187, 189, 192, 194, 198, 203, 209, 211, 214, 222, 225, 229, 231
power, 1, 2, 6, 7, 9, 11, 13–16, 19, 20, 51, 67, 69, 74, 75, 81, 83, 85, 86, 88–92, 95, 98, 104–107, 111, 117, 156–159, 169, 209–211, 218, 224, 228
practice, 10, 40, 171
precursor, 27
predator, 102

Index

pregnancy, 1–3, 5–13, 18, 25, 27, 28, 31, 33, 35, 36, 38, 41, 43, 45, 48, 49, 54, 55, 62, 64–67, 77, 78, 80, 83, 95, 98, 101, 110, 115–117, 121, 123–130, 132–135, 137–142, 145–148, 150, 153, 154, 156, 159, 161, 163, 166, 168, 169, 171, 174, 177, 178, 182–184, 187–189, 193, 196, 198, 212, 213, 217, 227
preparation, 132, 186
presence, 127
pressure, 66, 130, 140, 215
prevail, 77, 95
prevention, 127, 128
prey, 102
principle, 7, 177
priority, 124
privacy, 21, 43–45, 111, 176, 183, 184, 194
procedure, 74, 77, 79
process, 1, 3, 4, 10, 12, 15, 16, 18–20, 27, 30, 38–40, 46–48, 52, 74–78, 80, 81, 85, 93, 99, 106, 115, 117, 137, 144, 153, 170, 171, 179, 186, 189, 193, 205, 213, 216, 219, 225, 226, 231
processing, 138
procreation, 174
product, 183
production, 183
professional, 15, 74, 106, 138, 142, 183, 188, 213
profile, 45
progesterone, 137

progress, 5
projection, 187
prosperity, 5
protection, 18, 127, 215
protector, 91
provider, 91
psychology, 51, 112, 229
public, 125, 166–168, 174–179, 229
purpose, 51, 53, 67, 78, 85

quality, 49, 73, 132, 183
questionnaire, 29

race, 229
range, 55, 61, 74, 77, 80, 81, 89, 110, 117, 129, 138, 148, 172, 174, 185, 188
realism, 17, 52, 54, 62, 79, 84, 225
reality, 8, 85, 88, 90, 117, 137, 138, 140, 151–154, 174, 198–201, 212
realm, 1, 9, 10, 16, 25, 28, 33, 38, 41, 45, 48, 83, 101, 112, 128, 148, 156, 159, 169, 171, 187, 196, 198, 203, 206, 209, 212, 214
reassurance, 52, 117, 141
rebellion, 187
recovery, 70, 72, 137–139
redefinition, 187
reevaluation, 204, 205
reference, 216
reflection, 46, 117, 138, 153, 184, 214
rejection, 140
relationship, 15, 18, 22, 24, 25, 27, 45, 62, 64, 65, 94, 127, 141, 150, 153, 154, 156,

159, 163, 166, 169, 181, 184, 200, 210, 213, 215
relief, 138
reluctance, 229
reminder, 55, 101, 161
remorse, 154
René Descartes, 5
representation, 16, 183, 218, 219
repression, 5, 12
reproduction, 1–3, 5–7, 9, 10, 12, 41, 42, 49, 67, 69, 70, 77, 78, 81, 95, 98, 104, 129, 140, 154, 218, 224–226
requirement, 183
research, 18, 154, 227, 229
resentment, 113, 212
resilience, 43, 95
resonance, 78
resource, 195
respect, 11, 15, 16, 27, 28, 33, 93, 106, 109, 111, 117, 120, 123, 147, 168, 178, 179, 200, 211, 214, 215, 217, 219, 227
responsibility, 14, 154, 178
result, 217
reverence, 5
revolution, 5
rhythm, 100
richness, 224
rift, 212
right, 33, 95, 150, 178
rise, 2, 5, 6, 217
risk, 113, 115–117, 127, 128
rite, 7
ritual, 54, 106
role, 6, 15, 20, 48, 78, 80, 85, 91, 100, 102, 104, 106, 156, 158, 159, 179, 181, 183, 187, 196, 217, 218, 225, 226
roleplay, 1, 3–6, 8–11, 13–22, 27, 29, 30, 33–36, 38–40, 46, 50–59, 61–64, 70–75, 78–81, 83–86, 88–90, 93, 96, 97, 101–103, 106, 108, 110–112, 114, 117, 123–125, 127, 128, 130–134, 138, 140, 141, 144–146, 151, 153, 156, 161, 166, 167, 169, 176–179, 184, 193, 200, 203, 206, 208, 209, 211, 213, 214, 216
roleplaying, 50, 56–58, 62, 64, 67, 79, 80, 83, 124, 126, 138, 147, 166, 168, 183, 193, 200
rollercoaster, 18
routine, 127
rule, 45
rush, 12

safeguard, 183
safety, 3, 14, 17, 38, 56, 78, 85, 101, 117, 122–125, 127, 128, 130, 133, 140, 142, 163, 169, 171, 195, 196, 201, 211, 212, 214, 217–219
safeword, 10, 29, 128, 153, 161, 208, 216
sake, 130
Sam, 67
sanctity, 5
Sarah, 43
satisfaction, 169, 171
saturation, 183

Index

scenario, 3, 10, 15–21, 24, 27, 30, 48, 52, 58, 63, 64, 75, 78, 80, 86, 97, 106, 127, 128, 138, 141, 153, 161, 177, 178, 200, 210, 215
scene, 10, 17, 19, 20, 33, 36, 62, 111, 117, 177, 183, 208
science, 5, 17, 53
script, 190
secrecy, 141, 154, 218
section, 1, 9, 13, 22, 25, 28, 33, 36, 38, 41, 46, 48, 56, 65, 70, 78, 81, 83, 86, 88, 93, 101, 104, 107, 112, 115, 117, 123, 128, 130, 133, 135, 137, 139, 142, 145, 151, 156, 163, 166, 174, 176, 179, 184, 187, 193, 198, 203, 206, 209, 214, 222, 224, 227
security, 14, 21, 28, 45, 117, 166, 183
seduction, 54
selection, 77
self, 43, 46, 48, 67, 70, 98, 130, 137–139, 142, 150–154, 159–161, 184, 186, 187, 189, 201, 214, 216, 226, 231
sense, 3, 8, 14, 16–18, 21, 28, 51–55, 62, 67, 74, 75, 79, 85, 98, 106, 114, 130, 138, 153, 154, 161, 184, 189, 194, 195, 212, 214, 217, 224
sensitivity, 3, 6, 19, 77, 145, 171, 212, 218
sensuality, 188
series, 152, 218
seriousness, 21
session, 30, 141, 153, 161, 182, 200, 208
set, 17, 20, 29, 62, 145, 169, 176
setting, 15, 28–30, 79, 80, 142, 182, 188, 216, 225
sex, 2, 128, 184–187, 215, 217
sexual, 1, 2, 5–7, 9, 41, 43, 45, 48, 49, 54, 62, 65–67, 81, 83, 88, 102, 117, 127–129, 138, 140, 142, 149, 154, 173, 174, 181, 209, 212–214, 217–220, 225, 228, 229
sexuality, 1–3, 5–7, 9, 12, 41, 43, 70, 98, 102, 130, 138, 140, 154, 171, 173, 174, 177, 178, 184, 187, 188, 214, 217–219, 222, 224, 229
shame, 7, 111, 140, 141, 151, 154, 156, 174, 188, 217, 218
shaming, 194
shape, 5, 6, 9, 102, 137, 140, 214, 227
share, 6, 8, 109, 128, 156, 169, 193, 195, 200, 208, 217, 218, 227, 229
sharing, 43, 45, 98, 111, 136, 138, 182, 184, 194, 212
shift, 5, 67
shoot, 182
show, 218
Sigmund Freud, 6
Sigmund Freud's, 67, 102
sign, 148
signal, 10, 215
significance, 1, 9, 33, 36, 55, 117, 179, 190, 203
silence, 154

sire, 104
site, 187
size, 129
society, 5, 6, 98, 130, 141, 154, 174, 219
sociology, 229
software, 183
solace, 98
sound, 179
source, 7, 115, 174, 195
space, 12, 16, 19, 27, 34, 47, 55, 66, 75, 98, 117, 138, 141, 145, 147, 177, 179, 187, 193, 201, 206, 211–213
specific, 3, 30, 38, 54, 95, 102, 106, 124, 183, 187, 195
spectrum, 6, 52, 159, 176
sperm, 48, 49, 73, 77, 78, 99, 100, 225
spontaneity, 50, 63
stage, 62
staging, 183
standpoint, 145, 154
state, 7, 54, 129, 133
status, 128, 153
step, 12, 143, 148, 169, 171, 173, 213, 216
stigma, 2, 3, 7–9, 21, 41, 43, 77, 111, 140, 142, 171, 173–175, 188, 217, 218, 222, 227, 229
stillbirth, 145
stop, 10, 29, 33
storage, 183
storyline, 218
storytelling, 52, 83, 179, 181
strain, 213
strength, 19, 148
stress, 94

structure, 110
study, 187
style, 189
subject, 6, 147
submission, 7, 15, 20, 75, 85, 91, 92, 95, 102, 169, 183, 187
submissive, 14–16, 20, 75, 85, 91, 102, 107–109
subsection, 109
subset, 95
subversion, 187
success, 77, 225
summary, 6, 35
support, 19, 20, 22, 36, 38, 43, 48, 52, 65–67, 72, 80, 90, 95, 111, 118, 120, 125, 138, 141, 144, 148, 150, 156, 161, 172, 189, 194, 195, 213–217, 219, 227
surface, 16
surrender, 20, 75, 106
syringe, 128
system, 78, 98, 99, 121

taboo, 2, 6, 7, 11–13, 41, 111, 159, 163, 174, 217
talk, 161
tap, 17, 74, 81
tapestry, 21, 24, 53, 56, 67, 74, 106, 222
task, 171
Taylor, 45
teamwork, 67
technique, 73, 225
technology, 224–227
television, 218
temperature, 54
tenderness, 183
tension, 5, 140, 218

Index 249

term, 29
terrain, 109
territory, 198
test, 18
testing, 127, 128
theme, 51, 75, 182, 208
theory, 6, 12, 28, 67, 91, 102, 140, 151, 187
therapist, 66, 142, 149, 161, 213, 216
therapy, 142, 148–151, 153, 216
thought, 5, 179
thrill, 12, 15, 17, 18, 20, 49, 54, 56, 63, 81–83, 85, 140, 151, 154
time, 10, 25, 40, 43, 62–65, 111, 117, 153, 156, 195, 200, 216
timing, 15, 49, 54, 63, 73, 127
today, 193
toll, 94, 215
tool, 33, 70, 138, 193, 214
top, 124
topic, 6, 18, 20, 58, 77, 135, 218
touch, 18, 19, 30, 54, 169
tract, 78, 225
transformation, 5, 67, 70, 72
transition, 36, 111, 117, 141
transmission, 127
trauma, 213
treatment, 93–95
trigger, 75
trust, 15–17, 21, 24–27, 35, 38, 40, 45, 48, 49, 56, 74, 83, 85, 93, 97, 106, 107, 109, 123, 128, 132, 141, 166, 171, 206, 217
turbulence, 148
type, 13, 17, 19, 85, 123, 145

understanding, 1, 3, 5, 6, 9, 10, 13, 14, 16, 21, 27, 31, 38, 39, 41, 45, 51, 53, 56, 59, 62, 67, 72, 75, 77, 81, 85, 86, 88, 90, 93, 95, 98, 106, 109, 111, 112, 115, 117, 120, 123, 127, 130, 138, 141–143, 145, 147, 150, 151, 154, 156, 161, 163, 166, 168, 171, 173, 179, 184, 187, 189, 195, 200, 209, 212–214, 218, 219, 222, 224, 227, 229
unity, 54
unworthiness, 174
up, 19, 30, 53, 54, 62, 127
urgency, 54, 62, 63
use, 3, 10, 14, 17, 33–35, 78, 83, 86, 127, 128, 153, 161, 182, 194, 215, 225
uterus, 225

validation, 8, 21, 43, 98
variety, 17, 21, 51, 145
Venus, 5
vessel, 15
videography, 182–184
view, 8
vigilance, 211
violation, 164, 215
virtue, 5
visibility, 6, 178, 217, 219, 227
voice, 195
vulnerability, 1, 14, 15, 17, 19, 49, 52, 55, 67, 70, 74, 75, 81, 85, 86, 88, 106, 107, 115, 117, 154, 188, 228

warning, 214

warrant, 7
way, 6, 130, 171, 181, 187, 189, 211, 216, 226
weakness, 148
web, 2
weight, 19, 177
well, 15, 20, 31, 34–36, 38, 49, 54, 56, 75, 80–83, 93, 103, 121, 123, 125, 126, 134, 137, 139, 150, 151, 154, 156, 159, 194, 196, 214, 217–219, 227, 229

willingness, 53, 193, 206
window, 18, 49, 51, 54, 62–64, 183
withdrawal, 212
woman, 51, 62, 133, 225
word, 43, 153
work, 184, 210
workshop, 43
world, 19, 166, 168, 174
worry, 212
worship, 5
writing, 138

yoga, 66